Mathematics for Veterinary Medical Technicians
2nd Edition

Mathematics for Veterinary Medical Technicians

A Text/Workbook with Applications

Second Edition

Edward M. Stumpf

Frederick R. Fritz

William W. Bradford

Central Carolina Community College

Carolina Academic Press
Durham, NC

Copyright © 2006
Edward M. Stumpf, Frederick R. Fritz, and William W. Bradford
All Rights Reserved

Library of Congress Cataloging-in-Publication Data

Stumpf, Edward M.
  Mathematics for veterinary medical technicians : a text/workbook with applications / by Edward M. Stumpf, Frederick R. Fritz, William W. Bradford. -- 2nd ed.
    p.   cm.
   ISBN 1-59460-275-1
  1. Veterinary medicine--Mathematics--Handbooks, manuals, etc. I. Fritz, Frederick R. II. Bradford, William W. III. Title.

SF748.S78 2006
636.08901'51--dc22

2006018201

Carolina Academic Press
700 Kent Street
Durham, NC 27701
Telephone (919) 489-7486
Fax (919) 493-5668
www.cap-press.com

Printed in the United States of America

Contents

Introduction   vii

Acknowledgments   viii

Unit I

Chapter 1 – Roman Numerals   3

Chapter 2 – Introduction to Fractions   9

Chapter 3 – Multiplication and Division of Fractions   19

Chapter 4 – Addition and Subtraction of Fractions   35

Chapter 5 – Addition and Subtraction of Decimal Fractions   55

Chapter 6 – Multiplication and Division of Decimal Fractions   65

Fraction Review   87

Unit II

Chapter 7 – Percentage   93

Chapter 8 – Ratio and Proportion   115

Chapter 9 – Measurement Systems   129

Unit III

Chapter 10 – Dosage and Concentration Applications   161

Unit IV

    Chapter 11 – Diluting Concentrations and Infusion Rates   191

    Chapter 12 – Graphs and Graphing Techniques   209

Unit V

    Chapter 13 – Statistical Methods and Basic Statistics   227

Selected Solutions   239

Introduction

This text provides a one-semester course in the basics of mathematics needed for Veterinary Technicians and Assistants. The course covers fractions, decimals and percentage without the use of calculators as is the case on many State Board Exams. The language is designed to be readable and in terms of everyday usage rather than formal and strict mathematical terms.

This revised edition has used many of the suggestions for improvement that have been sent to us. Some material has been reordered to improve presentation.

In addition to basic mathematical computations, several chapters are devoted to application problems involving dosage, concentration, dilution and the computation of drip rates. The English, Metric and Avoirdupois systems of measurement are included with intra– and inter–system conversion and computation. An introduction to reading graphs is presented as well as a chapter on basic statistical concepts and using basic statistical measures.

The workbook style of the text allows students freedom to move at a pace that ensures mastery of the material as well as flexibility for covering topics in any prescribed manner. Students should read the material, study the examples, and work all the exercises in a particular problem set before checking answers. The answers to odd–numbered exercises are provided in the Answer Keys.

In many programs, this may be the only math course students are required to take. If this is one of your early course offerings, the material will be valuable and useful in other courses, in particular chemistry and clinical practices labs.

It is our hope that you will find the material useful and pertinent. If you have comments or suggestions please contact me at:

> Edward Stumpf
> Central Carolina Community College
> estumpf@cccc.edu

Acknowledgments

We would like to thank those who contributed in the writing and production of this text. In particular, Doctor Paul Porterfield, Lori Rainforth and the Veterinary Technology Department of Central Carolina Community College and all the Veterinary Medical students who used early versions of the text and offered suggestions for improvement and corrections.

Unit I

Chapter 1
Roman Numerals

Two systems of numeration are used by physicians and technicians – Arabic Numerals and Roman Numerals. The Arabic system utilizes the numerals 0, 1, 2, 3, 4, 5, 6, 7, 8, 9. It is the system most commonly used in all fields. All numerical values may be expressed by combinations of these ten symbols. The Arabic system is used to express weights and measures of the metric system and fractional units of the apothecaries' system.

The Roman system is sometimes used to indicate small quantities as well as being used in prescriptions. Roman numerals are encountered less often these days than in the past. Still, some knowledge of Roman numerals is desired of the technician. There are several simple rules governing Roman numerals.

Various Roman numerals in common use are:

Arabic	Roman
1	I or i
5	V or v
10	X or x
50	L or l
100	C
500	D
1000	M

In the Roman system, seven letters are used as symbols for numerals (indicated above). These letters are combined to express numerical values. When the apothecary system of measurement is used, whole units are expressed by Roman numerals. Lowercase or uppercase (capital) letters may be used to express Roman numerals, but it is customary to use small letters to indicate values of apothecary units. Cases are not mixed. Values over 30 are seldom used in medical practice. However, Roman numerals above 30 are encountered occasionally and the medical practitioner should be familiar with the rules governing their use. The lower-case Roman numeral i (1) is always written with a dot over it to avoid confusion with the lower-case Roman letter l (50). In modern times, the use of lowercase Roman numerals has declined for values of fifty or more, but are used more extensively for lesser values.

When reading or writing Roman numerals, pay attention to the position of the lesser values of numerals, such as I or V, in relation to the numerals of greater value, such as X or L.

Rules for Reading or Writing Roman Numerals

1) When a numeral is followed by the same numeral or by one of lesser value, the values of the numerals are added:

        ii or II   xiii or XIII   xv or XV

means 1 + 1 or 2   means 10 + 1 + 1 + 1 or 13   means 10 + 5 or 15

2) When a numeral is written before one of greater value, the lesser value is subtracted from the greater one.

        iv or IV   ix or IX

    means 5 – 1 or 4   means 10 – 1 or 9

3) When a numeral is written between two or more numerals of greater value, its value is subtracted from the sum of the others in the numeral.

        xix or XIX   xxxix or XXXIX

means 10 + 10 – 1 = 20 – 1 or 19   means 10 + 10 + 10 + 10 – 1 = 40 – 1 or 39

        xxiv or XXIV   XLIX

    10 + 10 + 5 –1 = 24   50 – 10 + 10 – 1 = 49

4) A single one, I (i) can precede only V (v) or X (x)

    iv = 4 or IX = 9 are okay

    IIX or IIL or IL are **not** okay.

A single X (x) can precede only L or C .

        XL for 40   or   XC for 90

A single value for 100, C, can precede only D or M

    CD = 400   CM = 900   CDXC = 490

5)   The numerals I (i), X (x), C and M are used a maximum of three times in succession. The numerals for 5 and 50, V (v) and L, respectively, are never used in succession.

    iii or III   xxx or XXX

means 1 + 1 + 1 is 3   means 10 + 10 + 10 = 30

Very large values use the same rules in the same order — the numbers are simply more complex. Look for such numbers during movie credits where they're often used for copyrights or film release dates.

        MCXXIV   MCMXXIV
M   C   XX   IV   M   CM   XX   IV
1000 + 100 + 20 + 4 =   1000 + 900 + 20 + 4 =
        1124   1924

        MCMXLIX   MMCMLXXXVIII
M   CM   XL   IX   MM   CM   LXXX   VIII
1000 + 900 + 40 + 9 =   2000 + 900 + 80 + 8 =
       1949   2988

Practice Set I - 1   Convert to Roman or Arabic numerals as appropriate

1. _____ XX
2. _____ MCLXXIX
3. _____ LXIV
4. _____ XXVI
5. _____ XCIX
6. _____ XXIII
7. _____ CDXLVIII
8. _____ xix
9. _____ MMMCCCXXXIII
10. _____ xxix
11. _____ iv
12. _____ CX
13. _____ III
14. _____ xxiv
15. _____ LVII
16. _____ CDIX
17. _____ xxxii

18. 15 _____
19. 1973 _____
20. 30 _____
21. 9 _____
22. 2435 _____
23. 29 _____
24. 112 _____
25. 49 _____
26. 8 _____
27. 2222 _____
28. 16 _____
29. 4 _____
30. 14 _____
31. 54 _____
32. 11 _____
33. 76 _____
34. 59 _____

Chapter 2
Introduction to Fractions

The actual measurement of many of the quantities with which we deal in the lab, in the home and in business force us to realize that the use of whole numbers alone is not sufficient to represent all information. We are simply compelled to use fractional measurements.

The parts of a fraction are called terms. In any common fraction there are two terms — the Numerator and the Denominator. The *Denominator* is the number written below the line of the fraction. It shows into how many equal parts the unit has been divided. In the following fractions, which number is the denominator:

$$\text{a. } \frac{2}{3} \quad \text{b. } \frac{3}{7} \quad \text{c. } \frac{2}{5} \quad \text{d. } \frac{1}{16}$$

If your answers are 3, 7, 5, 16, then you are correct.

Fraction "a" indicates a whole unit has been divided into how many equal parts? _____

If you selected 3, you are correct.

The *Numerator* is the number written above the line of the fraction and shows how many equal parts there are of the unit. In the following fractions, which number is the Numerator?

$$\text{a. } \frac{1}{16} \quad \text{b. } \frac{7}{12} \quad \text{c. } \frac{1}{2} \quad \text{d. } \frac{3}{8}$$

Your answers should read: 1, 7, 1, 3

10   Introduction to Fractions

The following figures have been divided into equal parts. A certain number of these parts have been shaded. Write the fraction that indicates what part of each figure is shaded.

(a)

(b)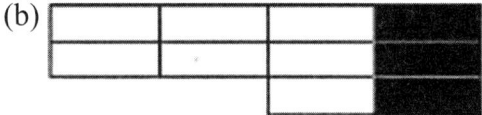

(c)

(d)

Your answer for "a" should be $1/2$. The denominator 2 indicates the units have been divided into two equal parts. The numerator 1 indicates that only one of the equal parts has been shaded. The correct answer for "b", "c", and "d" is $3/10$, $3/4$ and $5/6$, respectively.

Introduction to Fractions   11

In Practice Set II – 1 express your answers as fractions. Be sure to check your answers and correct errors.

Practice Set II - 1

1. List the shaded parts of each figure in terms of a fraction:

a.

b.

c.

d.

2. There are 12 inches in a foot. Express each of the following as a fraction of a foot:

    a. 1 in. _____   **b.** 5 in. _____   **c.** 11 in. _____   **d.** 7 in. _____

3. There are 36 inches in a yard. Express each of these as fractions of a yard:

    a. 1 in. _____   **b.** 35 in. _____   **c.** 13 in. _____   **d.** 19 in. _____

4. Express each of the following as fractions of an hour:

    a. 7 min. _____   **b.** 13 min. _____   **c.** 30 min. _____   **d.** 45 min. _____

5. Express each of the problems shown as fractions of a dollar:

    a. 12 cents _____   **b.** 37 cents _____   **c.** 50 cents _____   **d.** 99 cents _____

12 Introduction to Fractions

Common Fractions are fractions whose numerators and denominators are whole numbers.

Examples: (i) $\dfrac{1}{2}$ (ii) $\dfrac{16}{9}$ (iii) $\dfrac{2}{3}$ (iv) $\dfrac{5}{4}$

Proper Fractions are fractions which are less than one, that is whose numerators are less than the denominators.

Examples: (i) $\dfrac{1}{2}$ (ii) $\dfrac{1}{3}$ (iii) $\dfrac{16}{19}$ (iv) $\dfrac{8}{9}$

Improper Fractions have numerators which are equal to or larger than the denominators.

Examples: (i) $\dfrac{11}{6}$ (ii) $\dfrac{24}{23}$ (iii) $\dfrac{4}{3}$ (iv) $\dfrac{8}{5}$

Mixed Numbers are numbers composed of a whole number and a fraction.

Examples: (i) $1\dfrac{5}{6}$ (ii) $1\dfrac{1}{23}$ (iii) $1\dfrac{1}{3}$ (iv) $1\dfrac{3}{5}$

Notes:
(a) Improper fractions can be converted to mixed numbers and vice versa.
(b) The examples shown for improper fractions correspond in values to those shown for mixed numbers.

Complex fractions are usually "fractions over fractions"; or fractions or mixed numbers in the numerator or the denominator or both.

Examples: i. $\dfrac{\raise2pt{½}}{\raise-2pt{⅞}}$ ii. $\dfrac{\raise2pt{¾}}{\raise-2pt{²⁄₉}}$

Reducing fractions, or expressing fractions in lowest terms, is a general practice used everywhere. It makes fractions easier to read and understand.

Example: Which is easiest to understand and use?

$$\frac{1}{3} \text{ or } \frac{17}{51} \text{ or } \frac{34}{102}$$ They all have the same value.

In order for a fraction to be reduced to lowest terms, both the numerator and denominator must be divisible by the same number.

$\frac{5}{10}$ ← reduces to 1 when the numerator is divided by 5
← reduces to 2 when the denominator is divided by 5

$\frac{3}{12}$ ← divided by 3 = 1
← divided by 3 = 4

Note that the value of the fraction does not change.

$$\frac{5}{10} = \frac{1}{2} \qquad \frac{3}{12} = \frac{1}{4}$$

For the smaller fractions, the number used to divide is generally easy to determine.

Examples:

(i) $\dfrac{4 \;\; \text{divide by 4}}{8 \;\; \text{divide by 4}} = \dfrac{1}{2}$ (ii) $\dfrac{3 \;\; \text{divide by 3}}{9 \;\; \text{divide by 3}} = \dfrac{1}{3}$

However, when the number is larger, it can be more difficult to determine a single number that reduces both the numerator and denominator. Successive applications of the procedure can be used instead. The method remains the same and can be performed in multiple steps. First, find a number which will divide into both numerator and denominator. Then, inspect the resulting fraction to see if it can be further reduced.

Introduction to Fractions

Example: $\dfrac{16}{64} \left(\dfrac{\div 4}{\div 4}\right) = \dfrac{4}{16} \left(\dfrac{\div 4}{\div 4}\right) = \dfrac{1}{4}$

This example was performed in two steps. It could have been completed in one step if it had been observed that both numerator and denominator were divisible by 16.

$$\dfrac{16}{64} \left(\dfrac{\div 16}{\div 16}\right) = \dfrac{1}{4}$$

Some helpful hints are:
  (a) If both numbers are even, then they will be divisible by 2.
  (b) If the sum of the digits is divisible by 3, the number is divisible by 3.
  (c) If both numbers end in 0 or 5, then they are divisible by 5.

This is often a trial-and-error procedure until proficiency is acquired. A good knowledge of both multiplication and division tables is extremely helpful.

Practice Set II-2 Reduce each of the following fractions to the lowest terms:

1. $\dfrac{3}{5} =$ 2. $\dfrac{2}{4} =$ 3. $\dfrac{4}{8} =$ 4. $\dfrac{12}{16} =$

5. $\dfrac{12}{3} =$ 6. $\dfrac{9}{27} =$ 7. $\dfrac{13}{26} =$ 8. $\dfrac{21}{24} =$

9. $\dfrac{8}{9} =$ 10. $\dfrac{20}{30} =$ 11. $\dfrac{45}{81} =$ 12. $\dfrac{22}{77} =$

Improper Fractions and Mixed Numbers

To change improper fractions to mixed numbers, divide the denominator into the numerator for a whole number value. After dividing, the remainder becomes the numerator of the fraction. The denominator of the fraction is the same as the denominator of the improper fraction.

Examples:

(i) $\dfrac{7}{5}$ divide 5 into 7 which equals 1 with remainder of 2. This 2 becomes the numerator and the denominator stays at 5 $= 1\dfrac{2}{5}$

(ii) Convert $\dfrac{12}{5}$ to a mixed number.

$\dfrac{12}{5}$ divide 5 into 12 $5\overline{)12}\atop{\underline{-10}}\atop{2}$ (quotient 2) write the mixed number

determine the remainder (2) $= 2\dfrac{2}{5}$

(iii) $\dfrac{6}{5} \longrightarrow 5\overline{)6}\atop{\underline{5}}\atop{1}$ ← remainder $= 1\dfrac{1}{5}$

(iv) $\dfrac{19}{6} \longrightarrow 6\overline{)19}\atop{\underline{18}}\atop{1}$ = remainder $\longrightarrow = 3\dfrac{1}{6}$

(v) $\dfrac{18}{4} \longrightarrow 4\overline{)18}\atop{\underline{16}}\atop{2} \longrightarrow = 4\dfrac{2}{4} \longrightarrow = 4\dfrac{1}{2}$

divide rewrite reduce to lowest terms

Introduction to Fractions

To change mixed numbers to improper fractions, the whole number portion is multiplied by the denominator of the fraction. This new figure is then added to the original numerator and replaces it and the sum becomes the new numerator.

$2\frac{1}{3} \longrightarrow \frac{7}{3}$ 2 x 3 = 6 plus 1 is 7

add the numerator; multiply; denominator remains the same

Example: $3\frac{4}{5} = \frac{19}{5}$ 5 x 3 = 15; plus 4 is 19

denominator remains the same

Practice Set II - 3

Convert to a mixed number or an improper fraction as appropriate.

1. $\dfrac{10}{3} =$

2. $\dfrac{17}{5} =$

3. $\dfrac{25}{4} =$

4. $\dfrac{33}{8} =$

5. $\dfrac{35}{16} =$

6. $\dfrac{12}{3} =$

7. $4\dfrac{1}{3} =$

8. $16\dfrac{1}{2} =$

9. $1\dfrac{9}{10} =$

10. $5\dfrac{2}{7} =$

11. $3\dfrac{8}{9} =$

12. $12\dfrac{3}{4} =$

Practice Set II - 4

1. Reduce each fraction to lowest terms:

   a. $\dfrac{11}{44}$ b. $\dfrac{17}{102}$ c. $\dfrac{24}{25}$

   d. $\dfrac{12}{48}$ e. $\dfrac{48}{96}$ f. $\dfrac{5}{30}$

   g. $\dfrac{4}{32}$ h. $\dfrac{3}{27}$

2. Change to improper fractions:

   a. $8\dfrac{7}{8}$ b. $2\dfrac{13}{18}$ c. $7\dfrac{5}{6}$

   d. $3\dfrac{5}{8}$ e. $4\dfrac{11}{12}$ f. $7\dfrac{5}{7}$

   g. $6\dfrac{8}{9}$ h. $2\dfrac{5}{8}$

Introduction to Fractions

3. Change to mixed numbers:

a. $\dfrac{51}{17}$ b. $\dfrac{48}{7}$ c. $\dfrac{55}{9}$

d. $\dfrac{64}{9}$ e. $\dfrac{85}{4}$ f. $\dfrac{25}{7}$

g. $\dfrac{21}{5}$ h. $\dfrac{21}{4}$

Chapter 3
Multiplication and Division of Fractions

Multiplication of Fractions

Multiplication can be defined as successive addition. That is, $3 \times {}^1/_8$ means $\frac{1}{8} + \frac{1}{8} + \frac{1}{8}$ or ${}^3/_8$.

Example:

$6 \times {}^2/_3$ means $\quad \frac{2}{3} + \frac{2}{3} + \frac{2}{3} + \frac{2}{3} + \frac{2}{3} + \frac{2}{3} \quad$ or $\quad \frac{2}{3} + \frac{2}{3} + \frac{2}{3} + \frac{2}{3} + \frac{2}{3} + \frac{2}{3} = \frac{12}{3} = 4$

$\underbrace{\qquad\qquad\qquad}_{6 \text{ times}}$

Multiplication is a short cut for repeated addition and can be a time saver in the clinic. Notice in the examples given, we have been multiplying a whole number times a fraction. Fractions are multiplied across numerators and denominators. Since any whole number can be written with the numeral one (1) as a denominator, examine the following examples of multiplying fractions.

Examples: $\quad 4 \times \frac{2}{5} \quad$ is the same as $\quad \frac{4}{1} \times \frac{2}{5} \quad$ and $\quad \frac{2}{3} \times 5 = \frac{2}{3} \times \frac{5}{1}$

20   Multiplication and Division of Fractions

Example Multiplying:

$$\frac{4}{1} \times \frac{2}{5} = \frac{4 \times 2}{1 \times 5} = \frac{8}{5} = 1\frac{3}{5} \quad \textit{always reduce to lowest terms}$$

$$\frac{2}{3} \times 5 = \frac{2}{3} \times \frac{5}{1} = \frac{2 \times 5}{3 \times 1} = \frac{10}{3} = 3\frac{1}{3} \quad \text{which is the same as} \quad \frac{2}{3} + \frac{2}{3} + \frac{2}{3} + \frac{2}{3} + \frac{2}{3} = \frac{10}{3} = 3\frac{1}{3}$$

Practice Set III – 1

Multiply the following fractions and whole numbers:

1. $4 \times \frac{1}{3} =$
2. $5 \times \frac{1}{4} =$
3. $7 \times \frac{1}{2} =$
4. $18 \times \frac{2}{9} =$

5. $4 \times \frac{5}{7} =$
6. $5 \times \frac{1}{2} =$
7. $\frac{1}{3} \times 5 =$
8. $\frac{5}{6} \times 10 =$

Multiplying fractions by fractions is done in the same manner. Multiply numerator by numerator and denominator by denominator. Simplify.

Examples:

(i) $\frac{1}{3} \times \frac{1}{2} = \frac{1 \times 1}{3 \times 2} = \frac{1}{6}$ (ii) $\frac{4}{9} \times \frac{2}{5} = \frac{4 \times 2}{9 \times 5} = \frac{8}{45}$

Multiplication and Division of Fractions

Practice Set III – 2
Multiply the following fractions. Be sure to reduce where necessary.

1. $\dfrac{1}{3} \times \dfrac{1}{3} =$

2. $\dfrac{1}{4} \times \dfrac{1}{4} =$

3. $\dfrac{1}{3} \times \dfrac{1}{4} =$

4. $\dfrac{2}{9} \times \dfrac{2}{3} =$

5. $\dfrac{3}{4} \times \dfrac{2}{5} =$

6. $\dfrac{2}{5} \times \dfrac{3}{5} =$

7. $\dfrac{3}{4} \times \dfrac{5}{8} =$

8. $\dfrac{7}{8} \times \dfrac{3}{5} =$

Now, we're going to examine a short cut that can frequently be used when multiplying fractions. Sometimes we can divide a numerator and a denominator each by the same factor and thus simplify the multiplication. This process is referred to as cancellation, since we "cancel" one or more of the factors being multiplied. This simplifies the whole process. Unfortunately, the term cancellation can confuse students; furthermore, it is not a very good description of the math concepts that allow one to "cancel".

Cancellation gets its name from the mechanics of the process as well as the effect. But, we're not really "canceling" anything – or somehow performing math magic. Rather it is based upon the principle that any number divided by itself is 1. Also, a number multiplied by 1 remains the same number. Thus,

$$\dfrac{5}{6} \times \dfrac{6}{7} = \dfrac{5 \times \overbrace{6}^{=1}}{7 \times 6} = \dfrac{5}{7} \times 1 = \dfrac{5}{7}$$

As you can see, the sixes "cancel" each other; hence the term cancellation. The result is a way to "short-cut" multiplication of fractions.

$$\dfrac{5}{\cancel{6}} \times \dfrac{\cancel{6}}{7} = \dfrac{5}{7}$$

22 Multiplication and Division of Fractions

When can this technique be applied? Think of a bow tie. If the terms you wish to cancel are at any of the points (the darkened circles) on the bow tie, then cancellation will "work" as long as those points are connected by a line (as shown.)

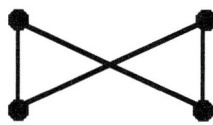

Here are some additional *examples:*

(i) $\dfrac{2}{\cancel{3}_1} \times \dfrac{\cancel{3}^1}{5} = \dfrac{2}{5}$

Threes connected

(ii) $\dfrac{3}{\cancel{4}_1} \times \dfrac{\cancel{8}^2}{11} = \dfrac{6}{11}$ since 4 goes into 4 one time and 4 goes into 8 two times

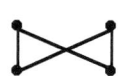

Four and eight lie at points connected by a line

(iii) $\dfrac{\cancel{5}^1}{\cancel{7}_1} \times \dfrac{\cancel{14}^2}{\cancel{25}_5} = \dfrac{2}{5}$

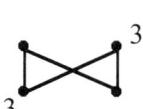

seven into 14 twice and 5 into 25 five times

(iv) $\dfrac{2}{3} \times \dfrac{2}{5} = \dfrac{4}{15}$ Remember the bow tie? The 2's won't cancel!

Multiplication and Division of Fractions

(v) $\dfrac{{}^2\cancel{4}}{7} \times \dfrac{3}{\underset{3}{\cancel{6}}} = \dfrac{6}{21} = \dfrac{2}{7}$ 2 divides into 4 two times and into 6 three times

$\dfrac{{}^2\cancel{4}}{7} \times \dfrac{\cancel{3}^1}{\underset{\underset{1}{\cancel{3}}}{\cancel{6}}} = \dfrac{2}{7}$ Same as above, but shown with the threes canceling each other; multiple cancellations are okay

(vi) $2 \times \dfrac{3}{8} \times \dfrac{6}{11}$

$\dfrac{{}^1\cancel{2}}{1} \times \dfrac{3}{\underset{\underset{2}{\cancel{8}}}{\cancel{8}}} \times \dfrac{\cancel{6}^3}{11}$ Multiple cancellations are allowed. Here, two divides evenly into itself and 8. It divides again into 4 and 6.

Multiply across numerators and denominators for the result.

$\dfrac{1}{1} \times \dfrac{3}{2} \times \dfrac{3}{11} = \dfrac{9}{22}$

Practice Set III – 3
Multiply each of the following. Use the "cancellation" technique wherever possible.

1. $\dfrac{4}{9} \times \dfrac{3}{5} =$
2. $\dfrac{2}{5} \times \dfrac{3}{10} =$
3. $\dfrac{2}{5} \times \dfrac{3}{8} =$
4. $\dfrac{4}{5} \times \dfrac{3}{10} =$

5. $\dfrac{3}{4} \times \dfrac{4}{5} =$
6. $\dfrac{9}{10} \times \dfrac{4}{27} =$
7. $\dfrac{2}{5} \times \dfrac{5}{8} =$
8. $\dfrac{5}{12} \times \dfrac{4}{15} =$

9. $\dfrac{3}{8} \times \dfrac{4}{9} =$
10. $\dfrac{7}{8} \times \dfrac{2}{7} =$
11. $\dfrac{2}{3} \times \dfrac{3}{4} \times \dfrac{12}{15} =$
12. $\dfrac{6}{7} \times \dfrac{14}{15} \times \dfrac{5}{8} =$

24 Multiplication and Division of Fractions

In the preceding sections, you have learned how to multiply fractions by whole numbers and whole numbers by fractions, how to multiply fractions by fractions and the technique of cancellation. Now, we'll learn how to multiply mixed numbers.

The only way to multiply mixed numbers is to first convert each mixed number to an improper fraction.

To multiply a mixed number by a whole number, change the mixed number to an improper fraction and multiply; cancel if possible; and reduce to lowest terms if possible.

Examples:

(i) $4\frac{2}{3} \times 9 = \frac{14}{3} \times 9 = \frac{14}{\cancel{3}} \times \frac{\cancel{9}^3}{1} = \frac{42}{1} = 42$

(ii) $3\frac{1}{2} \times 8 = \frac{7}{\cancel{2}} \times \frac{\cancel{8}^4}{1} = 28$

Practice Set III – 4
Multiply.

1. $5\frac{1}{3} \times 6 =$

2. $1\frac{1}{4} \times 4 =$

3. $8 \times 2\frac{3}{4} =$

4. $2 \times 5\frac{3}{4} =$

5. $6 \times 2\frac{1}{5} =$

6. $1\frac{2}{5} \times 3 =$

When both terms are mixed numbers change both mixed numbers to improper fractions and multiply.

Example: $4\dfrac{1}{8} \times 2\dfrac{2}{11} = \dfrac{\cancel{33}^{3}}{\cancel{8}_{1}} \times \dfrac{\cancel{24}^{3}}{\cancel{11}_{1}} = \dfrac{9}{1} = 9$

7. $2\dfrac{2}{3} \times 3\dfrac{1}{2} =$ 8. $3\dfrac{1}{3} \times 3\dfrac{2}{7} =$ 9. $4\dfrac{1}{5} \times 2\dfrac{1}{3} =$ 10. $7\dfrac{2}{3} \times 1\dfrac{1}{2} =$

11. $8\dfrac{1}{3} \times 6\dfrac{3}{4} =$ 12. $5\dfrac{1}{6} \times 2\dfrac{1}{2} =$ 13. $2\dfrac{3}{8} \times 3\dfrac{8}{16} =$ 14. $4\dfrac{1}{3} \times 3\dfrac{1}{4} =$

Applications: most of the problems you encounter in the working world are "word problems". That is, someone communicates information, verbally or written, and that information is used to solve some problem.

Practice Set III – 5

Solve the following application problems.

1. What is the total weight of 5 boxes each weighing 8 $1/4$ pounds?

2. Calculate the total weight of 12 steel cages if each cage is 11 feet long and each cage weighs 2 $1/8$ lb.. per foot.

3. What is the weight of 12 operating instruments, if each one weighs 1 3/4 pounds?

4. A gallon of a certain solution requires 5 7/8 ounces of a particular chemical. How many ounces of that chemical are needed to make three gallons of solution?

Division of Fractions

Draw a line 6 inches long like the one you see here.

_____

If you cut this line into 1/4 inch pieces, how many would you get? Mark it off and count them. You should have 24 vertical marks. Another way to find out the number of vertical marks needed is to divide 6 by 1/4.

Example:

$6 \div \dfrac{1}{4} =$ The number or fraction to the right is called the divisor. In this example 1/4 is the divisor.

$6 \times \dfrac{4}{1} =$ To divide by a fraction invert the divisor and multiply. (The answer is 24.)

When the numerator and denominator change places, we say the fraction has been *Inverted*. To invert means to turn over. A whole number like 5 when inverted becomes 1/5 therefore 1/5 is the *reciprocal* of 5. When dividing fractions, what we really do is multiply by the reciprocal.

Multiplication and Division of Fractions

Examples: The reciprocal of $\frac{1}{5}$ is 5.   The reciprocal of $\frac{2}{3}$ is $\frac{3}{2}$

$$3 \div \frac{1}{5} = \frac{3}{1} \times \frac{5}{1} = 15 \qquad 8 \div \frac{2}{3} = \frac{8}{1} \times \frac{3}{2} = 12$$

To divide fractions invert the divisor and multiply. If possible, reduce the result.

Examples: (i) $\frac{5}{6} \div \frac{5}{7}$

Divide fractions by inverting the divisor and multiplying. You may use cancellation techniques. Simplify if possible.

$$\frac{{}^1\cancel{5}}{6} \times \frac{7}{\cancel{5}_1} = \frac{7}{6} = 1\frac{1}{6}$$

(ii) $\frac{2}{3} \div \frac{1}{2}$

$$\frac{2}{3} \times \frac{2}{1} = \frac{4}{3} = 1\frac{1}{3}$$

(iii) $\frac{7}{12} \div \frac{3}{4}$ *or* $\frac{7}{12} \div \frac{3}{4}$

$$\frac{7}{\cancel{12}_3} \times \frac{\cancel{4}^1}{3} = \frac{7}{9} \qquad \frac{7}{12} \times \frac{4}{3} = \frac{28}{36} = \frac{7}{9}$$

Practice Set III – 6

Divide the following fractions.

1. $\frac{2}{3} \div \frac{4}{5} =$

2. $\frac{5}{16} \div \frac{5}{32} =$

3. $\frac{4}{5} \div \frac{2}{3} =$

4. $\frac{2}{9} \div \frac{3}{4} =$

5. $\frac{5}{12} \div \frac{3}{4} =$

6. $\frac{9}{16} \div \frac{3}{8} =$

7. $\frac{7}{8} \div \frac{5}{12} =$

8. $\frac{3}{16} \div \frac{9}{32} =$

Multiplication and Division of Fractions

Application:

9. A cafe owner used a 3/4 pound can of pepper to fill the pepper shakers. Each shaker can hold 1/64 pound of pepper. In this way, how many shakers would she fill from the 3/4 pound can?

Dividing a whole number by a fraction uses the same technique. Invert the divisor and multiply. It may be helpful to write the whole number as a fraction when you do this.

Examples: (i) $8 \div \dfrac{2}{5}$

$\dfrac{8}{1} \div \dfrac{2}{5}$

$\dfrac{8}{1} \times \dfrac{5}{2} = \dfrac{40}{2} = 20$

Write the whole number using 1 as a denominator. Invert the divisor and multiply. You may use cancellation if you desire.

(ii) $10 \div \dfrac{5}{7}$

$\dfrac{10}{1} \div \dfrac{5}{7}$

$\dfrac{\cancel{10}^{2}}{1} \times \dfrac{7}{\cancel{5}_{1}} = \dfrac{14}{1} = 14$

Practice Set III – 7

Solve.

1. $5 \div 1/3 =$

2. $4 \div \dfrac{1}{4} =$

3. $8 \div \dfrac{1}{2} =$

Multiplication and Division of Fractions

4. $25 \div \dfrac{5}{7} =$

5. $18 \div \dfrac{3}{4} =$

6. $45 \div {}^{9}/_{10} =$

7. $40 \div \dfrac{5}{8} =$

8. $96 \div \dfrac{24}{25} =$

9. $63 \div \dfrac{9}{10} =$

When dividing fractions by whole numbers, follow the same procedure. Make the divisor a fraction, then invert it and multiply.

Example:

$\dfrac{8}{9} \div 2 =$

$\dfrac{8}{9} \div \dfrac{2}{1} =$ Notice the use the reciprocal and multiplication.

$\dfrac{8}{9} \times \dfrac{1}{2} =$

$\dfrac{8}{18} = \dfrac{4}{9}$ Always reduce to lowest terms.

Practice Set III – 8
Divide.

1. $\dfrac{7}{8} \div 5 =$

2. $\dfrac{2}{3} \div 6 =$

3. $\dfrac{7}{16} \div 7 =$

4. $\dfrac{5}{8} \div 2 =$

5. $\dfrac{9}{11} \div 3 =$

6. $\dfrac{1}{4} \div 4 =$

Multiplication and Division of Fractions

When multiplying mixed numbers we first had to change any mixed numbers to improper fractions. The same procedure must be followed when dividing mixed numbers. To divide fractions involving mixed numbers change the mixed number to an improper fraction; invert the divisor, multiply, cancel where possible, reduce as necessary.

Examples:

(i) $3\frac{1}{2} \div 4$ change the mixed number to an improper fraction

$\frac{7}{2} \div 4$ change to multiplication and use the reciprocal of the divisor

$\frac{7}{2} \times \frac{1}{4} = \frac{7}{8}$

(ii) $5\frac{1}{3} \div 2\frac{2}{3}$ change mixed numbers to improper fractions

$\frac{16}{3} \div \frac{8}{3}$ invert the divisor and multiply

$\frac{16}{3} \times \frac{3}{8}$

$\frac{\cancel{16}^2}{\cancel{3}_1} \times \frac{\cancel{3}^1}{\cancel{8}_1} = \frac{2}{1} = 2$ multiply and simplify

Note the use of cancellation techniques.

Multiplication and Division of Fractions

Practice Set III – 9
Divide.

1. $6\dfrac{2}{3} \div \dfrac{1}{4} =$

2. $5\dfrac{3}{5} \div 7 =$

3. $4\dfrac{1}{3} \div 10 =$

4. $\dfrac{3}{5} \div \dfrac{9}{10} =$

5. $\dfrac{5}{8} \div 2\dfrac{1}{2} =$

6. $4\dfrac{1}{5} \div 1\dfrac{3}{4} =$

7. $30 \div 1\dfrac{2}{3} =$

8. $17\dfrac{1}{2} \div 3\dfrac{1}{2} =$

9. $6\dfrac{2}{5} \div 5\dfrac{1}{3} =$

10. $85 \div 4\dfrac{1}{4} =$

Practice Set III – 10
Review. Perform the indicated operation and simplify.

1. $\dfrac{7}{8} \times \dfrac{8}{9} =$

2. $1\dfrac{2}{3} \times \dfrac{3}{10} =$

3. $\dfrac{4}{5} \times \dfrac{1}{2} =$

4. $2 \times \dfrac{5}{8} \times 1\dfrac{3}{4} =$

5. $\dfrac{6}{8} \times \dfrac{2}{3} =$

6. $3\dfrac{1}{2} \times \dfrac{12}{8} \times 1\dfrac{1}{2} =$

Multiplication and Division of Fractions

7. $\dfrac{17}{51} \times \dfrac{1}{2} =$

8. $\dfrac{3}{3} \times \dfrac{2}{2} \times \dfrac{5}{5} =$

9. $\dfrac{9}{10} \times \dfrac{5}{3} =$

10. $\dfrac{1}{2} \div \dfrac{1}{4} =$

11. $\dfrac{9}{10} \times 1\dfrac{2}{3} =$

12. $\dfrac{1}{6} \div \dfrac{1}{8} =$

13. $1\dfrac{2}{3} \times 3\dfrac{1}{5} =$

14. $\dfrac{1}{3} \div \dfrac{2}{7} =$

15. $24 \times \dfrac{1}{2} =$

16. $1\dfrac{2}{5} \div \dfrac{3}{10} =$

17. $24 \times \dfrac{1}{3} =$

18. $2\dfrac{6}{10} \div \dfrac{10}{14} =$

19. $24 \times \dfrac{2}{3} =$

20. $8\dfrac{8}{10} \div \dfrac{11}{5} =$

21. $24 \times \dfrac{3}{3} =$

22. $2\dfrac{3}{4} \div \dfrac{11}{16} =$

23. $\dfrac{3}{4} \times \dfrac{2}{3} \times \dfrac{1}{2} =$

24. $3\dfrac{4}{5} \div 6\dfrac{7}{8} =$

Multiplication and Division of Fractions

25. $1\dfrac{2}{3} \div 4\dfrac{5}{6} =$

26. $9 \div \dfrac{1}{3} =$

27. $4 \div \dfrac{1}{2} =$

28. $\dfrac{1}{2} \div \dfrac{1}{4} =$

29. $\dfrac{2}{5} \div 1\dfrac{1}{4} =$

30. $\dfrac{8}{11} \div \dfrac{16}{22} =$

31. $4\dfrac{3}{5} \div \dfrac{23}{30} =$

32. $\dfrac{3}{3} \div \dfrac{2}{2} =$

33. $2\dfrac{1}{2} \div 2\dfrac{1}{2} =$

Chapter 4
Addition and Subtraction of Fractions

Addition of Fractions

Adding fractions with common denominators

To add or subtract fractions, a common denominator is required. To add fractions with a common denominator, add the numerators and write this sum over the common denominator.

Example:

$$\frac{1}{5} + \frac{2}{5} = \frac{1+2}{5} = \frac{3}{5}$$

(add the numerators; retain the common denominator)

The numerators 1 and 2 are added and their sum (3) is written over the common denominator (5). Reduce any fraction to lowest terms, if possible; and convert any improper fraction to a mixed number.

36   Addition and Subtraction of Fractions

Practice Set IV – 1

Add the following fractions. Be sure to reduce where necessary:

1. $\dfrac{3}{8} + \dfrac{4}{8} =$

2. $\dfrac{9}{16} + \dfrac{1}{16} =$

3. $\dfrac{3}{5} + \dfrac{1}{5} =$

4. $\begin{array}{r} \dfrac{7}{16} \\ + \dfrac{5}{16} \\ \hline \end{array}$

5. $\begin{array}{r} \dfrac{1}{7} \\ + \dfrac{2}{7} \\ \hline \end{array}$

6. $\begin{array}{r} \dfrac{5}{8} \\ \dfrac{1}{8} \\ + \dfrac{3}{8} \\ \hline \end{array}$

7. $\begin{array}{r} \dfrac{2}{16} \\ \dfrac{11}{16} \\ + \dfrac{7}{16} \\ \hline \end{array}$

Adding Fractions with Different Denominators

Fractions cannot be added unless they have a common denominator. Fractions have a common denominator when all their denominators are the same, as $\dfrac{5}{8}, \dfrac{7}{8}$, and $\dfrac{3}{8}$.

Example:

$$\dfrac{2}{3} + \dfrac{3}{4} + \dfrac{1}{2} = ?$$ Fractions without common denominators.

When the denominators are not the same, make them the same. First determine a common denominator, preferably, the **LCD** (*least common denominator*). That is, find the smallest number into which all the given denominators will divide evenly. In this example, the lowest number into which all the denominators (3, 4, and 2) will evenly divide is 12. This will be the least common denominator.

Addition and Subtraction of Fractions   37

The next step is to adjust the denominator in each fraction to a common denominator.

$$\frac{2}{3} \times \frac{}{4} = \frac{}{12}$$

$$\frac{3}{4} \times \frac{}{3} = \frac{}{12}$$

$$\frac{1}{2} \times \frac{}{6} = \frac{}{12}$$

by multiplying each denominator by a different number, we achieve the common denominator in each case

Then adjust the numerators in a similar fashion. Recall that any number multiplied by 1 is the same number – its value doesn't change. Furthermore, any fraction which has the same numerator and denominator is equal to 1. Since each denominator was multiplied by a different number in order to reach 12, multiply the numerators by that same number in each case.

$$\frac{2}{3} \times \frac{4}{4} = \frac{8}{12}$$

$$\frac{3}{4} \times \frac{3}{3} = \frac{9}{12}$$

$$\frac{1}{2} \times \frac{6}{6} = \frac{6}{12}$$

multiplying each fraction by the same number with which we achieved the denominator, adjusts the numerator.

We now have a common denominator and the fractions can be added.

Addition and Subtraction of Fractions

$$\frac{2}{3} \times \frac{4}{4} = \frac{8}{12}$$

$$\frac{3}{4} \times \frac{3}{3} = \frac{9}{12}$$

$$+ \frac{1}{2} \times \frac{6}{6} = \frac{6}{12}$$

$$\frac{23}{12}$$

Reduce to simplest form $\frac{23}{12} = 1\frac{11}{12}$

Another look at the same problem: $\frac{8}{12} + \frac{9}{12} + \frac{6}{12} = \frac{8+9+6}{12} = \frac{23}{12} = 1\frac{11}{12}$

Practice Set IV – 2

Add the fractions. Remember to find the LCD; reduce to simplest form where possible.

1. $\frac{1}{12} + \frac{1}{4} =$

2. $\frac{1}{6} + \frac{1}{3} =$

3. $\frac{1}{2} + \frac{1}{6} =$

4. $\frac{1}{4} + \frac{1}{2}$

5. $\frac{5}{12} + \frac{1}{4}$

6. $\frac{3}{8} + \frac{1}{4}$

7. $\dfrac{1}{8}$
   $+\dfrac{1}{2}$
   ─────

8. $\dfrac{3}{6}$
   $+\dfrac{1}{3}$
   ─────

9. $\dfrac{1}{8}$
   $+\dfrac{1}{4}$
   ─────

10. $\dfrac{1}{3}$
    $+\dfrac{1}{2}$
    ─────

11. $\dfrac{1}{7}+\dfrac{1}{2}=$

12. $\dfrac{3}{8}+\dfrac{3}{4}=$

13. $\dfrac{1}{16}$
    $\dfrac{1}{24}$
    $\dfrac{3}{48}$
    $+\dfrac{1}{6}$
    ─────

14. $\dfrac{1}{4}$
    $\dfrac{3}{8}$
    $\dfrac{3}{4}$
    $+\dfrac{5}{6}$
    ─────

15. $\dfrac{5}{6}$
    $\dfrac{1}{8}$
    $+\dfrac{2}{3}$
    ─────

Addition and Subtraction of Fractions

Here is a technique for finding the least common denominator. Suppose the problems has denominators of 6, 8 and 10. Using division without remainder, that is, divide evenly:

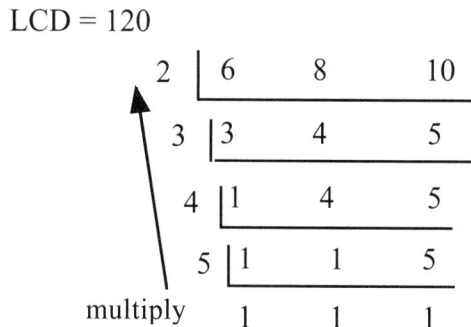

LCD = 120

Divide by any number that will divide evenly into any of the denominators. If it will not divide evenly, don't divide at all. The goal is to get all "1"s along the bottom row. You can see that first our denominators were divided by 2, followed by 3. This left a 1, 4 and 5.

Continue to divide using values that divide with no remainders. Once all 1s have been achieved along the bottom row, multiply up the "ladder" to find the LCD. In this case, it's 5 x 4 x 3 x 2 = 120.

Example: Denominators are 6, 14 and 5.

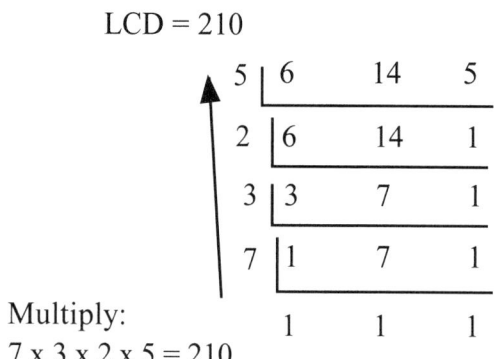

LCD = 210

Multiply:
7 x 3 x 2 x 5 = 210

Divide. Continue the process until the last row contains only 1s. Then multiply the numbers along the left side.

Adding Mixed Numbers

A mixed number is a number composed of a whole number and a fraction taken together, such as $3\frac{2}{5}$ or $1\frac{2}{3}$. To add mixed numbers — add the whole numbers and the fractions separately and combine the results. (*It is not necessary to convert to improper fractions as when multiplying or dividing.*) Simplify and reduce as needed.

Example:

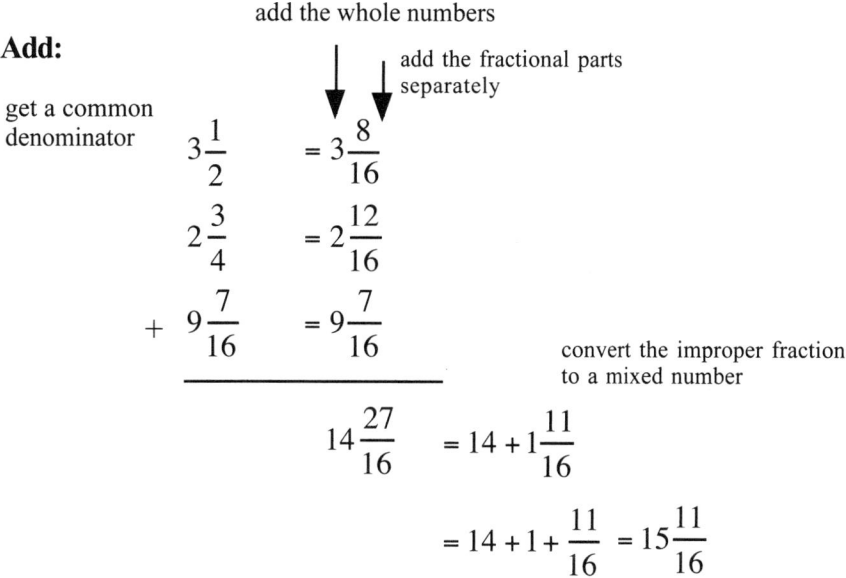

In this example, the fractions were changed to 16ths (for a common denominator) and added for a sum of $\frac{27}{16}$, which simplifies to $1\frac{11}{16}$. The sum of the whole numbers was 14. Combining these results yields the solution $15\frac{11}{16}$.

Another procedure for adding mixed numbers involves changing all the mixed numbers to improper fractions before adding. That procedure, while correct, tends to involve more steps thus increasing the possibility for error. If you know how to do this procedure, and are comfortable with doing it, then you are welcome to do so. In math, there are often several ways to a solution. Rarely, though, is there only one "right" way. Any method that is mathematically sound and achieves the desired result is acceptable.

Practice Set IV – 3

Add.

1. $5\dfrac{1}{3}$
   $+\,8\dfrac{1}{12}$

2. $4\dfrac{3}{5}$
   $+\,6\dfrac{1}{10}$

3. $7\dfrac{1}{2}$
   $+\,12\dfrac{1}{8}$

4. $8\dfrac{3}{10}$
   $+\,9\dfrac{2}{5}$

5. $8\dfrac{1}{2}$
   $+\,7\dfrac{1}{4}$

6. $14\dfrac{1}{6}$
   $+\,6\dfrac{1}{3}$

7. $15\dfrac{1}{10}$
   $+\,7\dfrac{1}{2}$

8. $9\dfrac{3}{8}$
   $+\,8\dfrac{1}{4}$

9. $6\dfrac{6}{16}$
   $+\,7\dfrac{1}{8}$

Addition and Subtraction of Fractions

10. $12\dfrac{1}{4}$
    $+\ 7\dfrac{1}{12}$
    _____

11. $6\dfrac{7}{10}$
    $+\ 8\dfrac{4}{5}$
    _____

12. $4\dfrac{3}{5}$
    $+\ 7\dfrac{11}{15}$
    _____

13. $9\dfrac{5}{6}$
    $+\ 6\dfrac{2}{3}$
    _____

14. $7\dfrac{1}{2}$
    $+\ 9\dfrac{3}{8}$
    _____

15. $3\dfrac{1}{9}$
    $+\ 5\dfrac{2}{3}$
    _____

Adding Improper Fractions

Improper fractions can be added in two ways: (1) Convert the improper fraction(s) to mixed numbers and add as previously shown; or (2) Determine the common denominator, add the fractions and then convert the answer to a mixed number.

Example:

$$\dfrac{3}{2} = \dfrac{9}{6}$$

$$\dfrac{5}{3} = \dfrac{10}{6}$$

$$+\ \dfrac{7}{6} = \dfrac{7}{6}$$

Determine LCD, adjust numerators and add

$$\dfrac{26}{6} = 4\dfrac{2}{6} = 4\dfrac{1}{3}$$

Convert to mixed number and reduce to lowest terms

Addition and Subtraction of Fractions

Practice Set IV – 4

Add the following.

1. $\dfrac{17}{16}$
    $\dfrac{9}{8}$
    $+\dfrac{3}{2}$

2. $\dfrac{3}{2}$
    $\dfrac{5}{4}$
    $+\dfrac{11}{8}$

3. $\dfrac{7}{5}$
    $\dfrac{9}{4}$
    $+\dfrac{12}{10}$

4. $\dfrac{27}{9}$
    $\dfrac{24}{8}$
    $+\dfrac{3}{2}$

Combinations of mixed numbers, whole numbers, and fractions — common and improper — are combined similarly.

Example: Sum. $\dfrac{2}{3} + 7 + 4\dfrac{1}{5} + \dfrac{7}{2} =$

$\dfrac{2}{3} = \dfrac{20}{30}$
$+ 7 = 7$ Determine common denominator.
$+ 4\dfrac{1}{5} = 4\dfrac{6}{30}$ Sum and simplify.
$+ \dfrac{7}{2} = \dfrac{105}{30}$

$11\dfrac{131}{30} = 11 + 4\dfrac{11}{30} = 15\dfrac{11}{30}$

Practice Set IV – 5

Add the following.

1. $1\frac{3}{4}$
   $\frac{5}{3}$
   $+\frac{1}{2}$

2. $4\frac{3}{5}$
   $6\frac{3}{8}$
   $+\frac{23}{20}$

3. $2\frac{1}{2}$
   $3\frac{1}{2}$
   $+2\frac{2}{3}$

4. $4\frac{3}{16}$
   $3\frac{2}{5}$
   $2\frac{1}{4}$
   $+1\frac{1}{2}$

Subtraction of Fractions

Subtracting fractions is very similar to adding fractions except now the arithmetic operation is subtraction. Nearly everything else you've learned about adding fractions applies to subtracting them as well.

To subtract proper fractions with like denominators, subtract the numerators and place the result over the common denominator. Remember to reduce or simplify if possible.

Example:

Vertically
$\frac{9}{16}$
$-\frac{7}{16}$
$\frac{2}{16} = \frac{1}{8}$

Or Horizontally

$\frac{9}{16} - \frac{7}{16} = \frac{9-7}{16} = \frac{2}{16} = \frac{1}{8}$

Addition and Subtraction of Fractions

Practice Set IV – 6

Subtract the following fractions with like denominators.

1. $$\frac{2}{3}$$
   $$-\frac{1}{3}$$

2. $$\frac{5}{6}$$
   $$-\frac{4}{6}$$

3. $$\frac{8}{11}$$
   $$-\frac{1}{11}$$

4. $$\frac{13}{16}$$
   $$-\frac{5}{16}$$

When subtracting fractions with unlike denominators, first determine a common denominator, then adjust the numerators as needed and subtract. This is exactly as you have done when adding fractions.

Examples:

$$\frac{5}{8} = \frac{5}{8}$$
$$-\frac{1}{4} = -\frac{2}{8}$$
$$\overline{}$$
$$\frac{3}{8}$$

$$\frac{7}{9} = \frac{7}{9}$$
$$-\frac{2}{3} = -\frac{6}{9}$$
$$\overline{}$$
$$\frac{1}{9}$$

Practice Set IV – 7
Subtract.

1. $\dfrac{3}{4} - \dfrac{3}{8}$

2. $\dfrac{5}{8} - \dfrac{1}{2}$

3. $\dfrac{1}{3} - \dfrac{1}{6}$

4. $\dfrac{1}{2} - \dfrac{3}{16}$

5. $\dfrac{15}{32} - \dfrac{1}{4}$

6. $\dfrac{1}{16} - \dfrac{1}{32}$

7. $\dfrac{17}{20} - \dfrac{1}{2}$

8. $\dfrac{9}{15} - \dfrac{1}{3}$

9. $\dfrac{11}{10} - \dfrac{1}{2}$

10. $\dfrac{16}{12} - \dfrac{1}{2}$

11. $\dfrac{12}{10} - \dfrac{1}{5}$

12. $\dfrac{12}{9} - \dfrac{1}{3}$

Addition and Subtraction of Fractions

Subtracting Mixed Numbers

Subtract mixed numbers just as you added them — subtract the fractions, then subtract the whole numbers.

Example:

$$11\frac{5}{6} = 11\frac{10}{12}$$
$$-3\frac{3}{4} = -3\frac{9}{12}$$
$$\overline{}$$
$$8\frac{1}{12}$$

Determine the LCD and convert the fractions

$$\frac{10}{12} - \frac{9}{12} = \frac{1}{12}$$

and

$$11 - 3 = 8$$

Practice Set IV – 8

Subtract these mixed numbers. Be sure to reduce to lowest terms where possible.

1. $7\frac{5}{8}$
   $-4\frac{1}{4}$

2. $9\frac{5}{8}$
   $-5\frac{1}{2}$

3. $15\frac{3}{4}$
   $-11\frac{1}{2}$

4. $8\frac{3}{4}$
   $-5\frac{5}{8}$

5. $13\frac{11}{18}$
   $-12\frac{4}{9}$

6. $10\frac{2}{5}$
   $-3\frac{1}{4}$

7. $9\frac{3}{4}$
   $-\frac{2}{3}$

8. $62\frac{7}{10}$
   $-50\frac{7}{20}$

9. $6\frac{2}{3}$
   $-3\frac{1}{5}$

10. $14\frac{1}{2}$
    $-2\frac{1}{4}$

Subtracting mixed numbers where the subtrahend is a larger fraction

Example:

$$2\frac{1}{4}$$ Minuend - the number from which another is being subtracted

$$-\frac{3}{4}$$ Subtrahend - the number which is subtracted

Note that we wish to subtract $\frac{3}{4}$ from $\frac{1}{4}$. But $\frac{3}{4}$ is larger than $\frac{1}{4}$.

This procedure can only be completed by "borrowing". Borrow a whole number (1), change it into a fraction and add it to the minuend; then subtract.

Example: Borrow one from the two, convert to a fraction ($1 = \frac{4}{4}$), then subtract. Reduce if possible.

$$
\begin{array}{cccccc}
2\frac{1}{4} & = 1 + 1\frac{1}{4} & = & 1 + \frac{4}{4} + \frac{1}{4} & = & 1\frac{5}{4} \\
-\frac{3}{4} & = -\frac{3}{4} & = & \phantom{1+\frac{4}{4}+}-\frac{3}{4} & = & -\frac{3}{4} \\
\hline
& & & & & 1\frac{2}{4} = 1\frac{1}{2}
\end{array}
$$

Addition and Subtraction of Fractions

Here is the same problem done another way and using a short cut.

$$\begin{array}{r} \overset{1}{\cancel{2}}\overset{1}{\tfrac{1}{4}} \\ -\tfrac{3}{4} \\ \hline \end{array}$$ borrow 1(whole unit) from the 2

$$\begin{array}{r} \overset{1}{\cancel{2}}\overset{5}{\cancel{\tfrac{1}{4}}} \\ -\tfrac{3}{4} \\ \hline \end{array}$$ add the numerator and denominator together creating a new numerator

$$\begin{array}{r} 1\tfrac{5}{4} \\ -\tfrac{3}{4} \\ \hline 1\tfrac{2}{4} = 1\tfrac{1}{2} \end{array}$$

this is the new Minuend

subtract and reduce

In practical terms, all you have to remember is to add the numerator and denominator (as in the first example) after you borrow. This works (as shown in detail in the second example) because any number over itself (that is, any time the numerator and denominator are the same) is equal to one. So if you borrow one whole number it will equal the same number of parts in which the fraction is represented.

Addition and Subtraction of Fractions

If unlike denominators are represented, first determine the common denominator, then borrow and subtract. Here's an *example* ...

$$3\frac{1}{5}$$
$$-1\frac{2}{3}$$
determine the LCD

$$3\frac{3}{15}$$
$$-1\frac{10}{15}$$

borrow
$$2\cancel{3}\frac{18}{15}$$
$$-1\frac{10}{15}$$
Add the numerator and denominator

$$2\frac{18}{15}$$
$$-1\frac{10}{15}$$
Subtract

$$1\frac{8}{15}$$

Practice Set IV – 9

Subtract the following mixed numbers:

1. $3\frac{2}{5}$
    $-2\frac{2}{3}$

2. $4\frac{3}{4}$
    $-1\frac{7}{8}$

3. $2\frac{1}{3}$
    $-\frac{5}{6}$

4. $1\frac{3}{4}$
    $-\frac{7}{8}$

5. $2\frac{3}{11}$
    $-\frac{7}{22}$

6. 16
    $-\frac{1}{2}$

7. 8
    $-\frac{4}{5}$

8. $1\frac{4}{9}$
    $-\frac{13}{18}$

9. $1\frac{9}{20}$
    $-\frac{4}{5}$

10. 9
    $-\frac{9}{16}$

Subtracting Improper Fractions

Except for the operation (subtraction), the techniques for subtracting are the same as for addition of improper fractions.

Examples:

(i) $\dfrac{11}{8} - \dfrac{9}{8} = \dfrac{2}{8} = \dfrac{1}{4}$

(ii) $\dfrac{16}{4} = \dfrac{32}{8}$ Determine the LCD

$-\dfrac{3}{8} = -\dfrac{3}{8}$ Subtract

$\dfrac{29}{8} = 3\dfrac{5}{8}$ Convert to mixed number; reduce if necessary

Practice Set IV – 10

Subtract the following:

1. $\dfrac{11}{9} - \dfrac{10}{9}$

2. $\dfrac{11}{9} - \dfrac{4}{18}$

3. $\dfrac{5}{4} - \dfrac{6}{5}$

4. $\dfrac{6}{5} - \dfrac{7}{6}$

5. $\dfrac{51}{18} - \dfrac{1}{9}$

Practice Set IV – Chapter Review

Solve each of the following:

1. $\dfrac{11}{17} + \dfrac{8}{34} =$

2. $1\dfrac{11}{17} - \dfrac{8}{34} =$

3. $\dfrac{1}{8} + \dfrac{1}{16} + \dfrac{3}{2} =$

4. $4\dfrac{1}{9} + 6\dfrac{11}{18} + 9\dfrac{1}{3} =$

5. $\dfrac{6}{8} - \dfrac{3}{5} =$

6. $4\dfrac{1}{8} - 1\dfrac{5}{7} =$

7. $1\dfrac{1}{2} + 2\dfrac{2}{3} + 3\dfrac{3}{4} + 4\dfrac{4}{5} =$

8. $4\dfrac{3}{4} - 3\dfrac{4}{5} =$

9. $4\dfrac{7}{8} - 2\dfrac{8}{9} =$

10. $6\dfrac{2}{3} - \dfrac{3}{4} =$

11. $1\dfrac{16}{17} - \dfrac{32}{34} =$

12. $\dfrac{7}{8} - \dfrac{2}{3} =$

13. $14\dfrac{5}{12} - 6\dfrac{9}{10} =$

14. $8\dfrac{3}{5} - \dfrac{7}{10} =$

15. $1\dfrac{5}{24} - \dfrac{1}{4} =$

Addition and Subtraction of Fractions

16. $\dfrac{2}{3} - \dfrac{2}{6} =$

17. $1\dfrac{4}{9} - \dfrac{5}{18} =$

18. $4\dfrac{1}{3} - \dfrac{4}{9} =$

19. $4\dfrac{2}{7} + \dfrac{1}{2} =$

20. $8 - \dfrac{4}{9} =$

21. $18\dfrac{1}{24} + 1\dfrac{7}{8} =$

22. $\dfrac{1}{3} - \dfrac{1}{8} =$

23. $\dfrac{4}{16} - \dfrac{1}{4} =$

24. $7\dfrac{1}{4} + \dfrac{2}{3} =$

Chapter 5
Addition and Subtraction of Decimal Fractions

In the first few chapters we studied the four operations of common fractions. Now we study a different fraction that is very important and has everyday applications in the clinic and at the lab. The new fraction to be studied in this section is the decimal fraction. A *decimal fraction* may be considered a common fraction whose denominator is 10 (or some power of 10), such as denominators of 100, 1,000 and so on.

Examples: $\dfrac{3}{10}$ can be written 0.3

$\dfrac{21}{100}$ can be written 0.21

$\dfrac{297}{1000}$ can be written 0.297

It is conventional to use a zero as the ones placeholder before the decimal to avoid any confusion and to point out that a decimal fraction follows.

Decimal Fractions

```
         .  | Decimal Point
            | Tenths
            | Hundredths
            | Thousandths
            | Ten-Thousandths
            | Hundred-Thousandths
            | Etc.
```

All numbers to the left of the decimal point are *whole numbers.*

In the chart, notice that one place to the right of the decimal point is tenths; two places to the right of the decimal point is hundredths, three places thousandths, and so forth. When reading the decimal point we say "and".

Example: 2.57   is read   two *and* fifty-seven hundredths

An alternate method involves the words "decimal" or "point" and read the numerals as:

2.57 reads as two point five seven   or   two decimal fifty-seven

When writing (or reading) decimals of small values, less than one for example, zeros are placed between the decimal point and the number in the decimal (if necessary).

Examples: seven hundredths is written   0.07
              nine thousandths   0.009

Practice Set V – 1
Write the following as decimal fractions.

1. nine tenths =

2. three tenths =

3. twenty-five hundredths =

4. nine ten-thousandths =

5. twelve thousandths =

6. twenty-two thousandths of an inch =

7. five tenths feet =

8. thirty-two thousandths =

Remember, decimals are really fractions, or parts, of a whole. We often use decimal representation instead of common fractions because decimal fractions can be simpler since they're based on powers of ten. We can easily change common fractions to decimal fractions by dividing the numerator by the denominator.

Example: Change $\frac{5}{8}$ to a decimal fraction.

$$\begin{array}{r}0.625\\8\overline{)5.000}\end{array}$$

Divide 5 by 8. Since 8 does not evenly divide into 5, we place the decimal point after the 5 (in the dividend), and immediately above that in the answer (the quotient). Annex zeros to the dividend and complete the division.

Decimal Fractions

To convert a mixed number to a decimal, keep the whole number and convert the fractional part to a decimal as in the previous example.

$$1\frac{3}{4} = 1.75 \qquad \text{since} \quad 4\overline{)3.00} = 0.75$$

Practice Set V – 2

Change the following common fractions to decimal fractions.

1. $\dfrac{11}{64}$
2. $\dfrac{3}{32}$
3. $\dfrac{5}{8}$
4. $\dfrac{5}{16}$
5. $\dfrac{1}{4}$

6. $\dfrac{1}{8}$
7. $\dfrac{5}{64}$
8. $\dfrac{1}{2}$
9. $1\dfrac{3}{8}$
10. $1\dfrac{7}{16}$

11. $\dfrac{3}{4}$
12. $\dfrac{7}{8}$
13. $2\dfrac{5}{8}$
14. $\dfrac{3}{80}$
15. $1\dfrac{9}{64}$

Decimal Fractions 59

To change decimal fractions to common fractions:

Example: change .45 to a common fraction.

$$.45 = \frac{45}{100} = \frac{9}{20} \text{ (reduced)}$$

decimal fraction   common fractions

Write the decimal, without the decimal point, over the appropriate tens units. Here, since the decimal is 45 hundredths, write 45 over 100.

Tip: count the decimal places and that indicates the number of zeros for the denominator.

Examples: (i) $0.456 = \dfrac{456}{1000}$ (ii) $0.0076 = \dfrac{76}{10,000}$

three decimal places, thus three zeros

four decimal places, thus four zeros

Practice Set V – 3
Change each of the following to common fractions and reduce to lowest terms.

1. 0.06
2. 0.250
3. 0.495
4. 0.33
5. 0.630

6. 0.009
7. 0.3
8. 0.3755
9. 1.188
10. 0.40

Rounding Decimals

Sometimes, it is necessary to express an answer correct to the nearest hundredth or to the nearest thousandth, for example. After finding the solution, the answer may be rewritten with as many decimal places as are required to bring it to the degree of accuracy determined by the problem. This process is known as rounding off a number. Rounding off means expressing a decimal with fewer digits. The answer should be determined to one more place than the accuracy calls for, then "rounded" as indicated by that digit. Round to the nearest hundredth means the answer should have two decimal places. Thus, the answer should be carried to three places and the answer rounded off to two places. If the digit to the right of the place we are rounding is 5 or more, drop it and add one to the digit in the place immediately to the left. If the digit is less than 5, drop it and do not change digit to its left.

Example: Round 0.671 to the nearest hundredth. Since the third decimal place (thousandths) is a 1, drop that and do not change the preceding digit (the 7) – the answer is then 0.67.

Round 0.876 to the nearest hundredth.

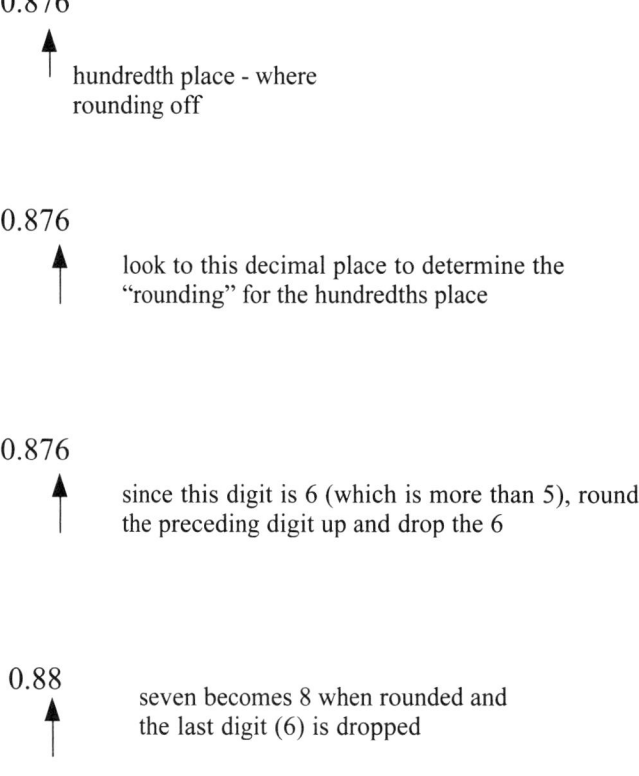

0.876 rounded to the nearest hundredth is 0.88

Decimal Fractions

You try it! Round 0.7536 to the nearest thousandth.   *(answer: 0.754)*

Practice Set V – 4

Round each of the following to the nearest 0.001

1. 0.8731   **2.** 0.7899   **3.** 0.7777

4. 0.6312   **5.** 0.6214   **6.** 0.7325

Round each of the following to the nearest 0.01

7. 0.654   **8.** 0.667   **9.** 0.372

10. 0.982   **11.** 0.427   **12.** 0.635

Round to the indicated (by underline) place.

13. 5_8_9   **14.** 0.003_2_9   **15.** 17_5_9

16. 0._8_428   **17.** 1_6_07   **18.** 0.8_5_49

19. 19_0_5   **20.** 0._0_02   **21.** 10_6_6

22. 1.9_8_08   **23.** _5_1   **24.** 4._5_49

25. 14_3_2   **26.** 1.4_3_2   **27.** 876_9_29

Decimal Fractions

Addition of Decimals

You already know how to add dollars and cents. Add all decimals the same way! The key to remember is to align the decimal points in a column. Add just as you would for whole numbers, placing the decimal point in the answer directly below the column of decimal points.

Example: Add.   6.25 + 21.021 + 873.0725 + 647

```
   6.25
  21.021
 873.0725
 647.
```
a common error involves "forgetting" that the decimal in a whole number belongs at the right end of that number

Some students like to even the columns using zeros in those numbers with fewer places so everything "lines up". Like this:

```
    6.2500
   21.0210
  873.0725
  647.0000
 ─────────
 1547.3435
```

Practice Set V – 4

Add the following.

1. 0.008, 20, 0.6, 4.5

2. 0.03, 0.3, 4.12, 30

3. 10, 0.0615, 1.2

4. 52.2, 0.06, 0.0008, 2000

5. 0.005, 2.5, 1.1

6. 0.006, 5, 0.32, 0.08

7. 0.05, 10.256, 12.2

8. 0.09, 10, 4.8, 1000

9. 0.05, 0.006, 0.032, 0.0003

10. 2.5, 1.98, 100, 0.8

11. 1.2, 1.5, 0.03, 15

12. 0.15, 0.4, 0.048, 6

13. 0.8, 1.5, 0.5

14. 0.64, 8, 0.06, 0.3

Subtraction of Decimals

Subtraction of decimals in done in the same manner. Align the decimal points, subtract, place the decimal in the answer directly in the same column place as each of the decimals. Again, you may add zeros so that all numbers align.

Example: subtract 15.275 from 32.63

$$
\begin{array}{r} 32.63 \\ -15.275 \\ \hline 17.355 \end{array}
\qquad
\begin{array}{r} 32.630 \\ -15.275 \\ \hline 17.355 \end{array}
$$

Decimal Fractions

Practice Set V – 5

Subtract.

1. 92.12 minus 0.37

2. 1,000 minus 810.77

3. 11,246.51 minus 247.59

4. 53.36 minus 43.65

5. 0.0257 from 9.3126

6. 4.695 from 7.342

7. 0.079 from 0.1032

8. 0.65832 from 1

Chapter 6

Multiplication and Division of Decimal Fractions

Multiplication of Decimals

In the previous chapter you learned how to add and subtract with decimals. In this section, we learn how to multiply and divide with decimals.

When multiplying numbers, the result, or answer, is called the product. The numbers being multiplied are called factors.

Examples: $5 \times 15 = 75$ The product is 75. The factors are 5 and 15.

$\dfrac{1}{2} \times \dfrac{2}{3} = \dfrac{2}{6} = \dfrac{1}{3}$ The product is $1/3$. The factors are $1/2$ and $2/3$.

$0.3 \times 0.5 = .15$ The product is 0.15. The factors are 0.3 and 0.5.

In the examples shown, it doesn't matter if the numbers are whole numbers, common fractions, or decimal fractions – the answer is called the product in each case of multiplication.

When multiplying decimals, proceed as in multiplying whole numbers. The process is the same. The only change is placing the decimal point in the proper position in the resultant product. Count the number of decimal places in each of the numbers multiplied. Place the decimal to the right of the product, as if it was a whole number, and move the decimal point one place to the left for each decimal place in the factors.

Example: $\begin{array}{r} 5 \\ \times\, 0.12 \\ \hline \end{array}$ How many decimal places are there? _____

Decimal Fractions

Your answer should have two decimal places for the two places in the factor 0.12. In the product start with the rightmost digit and move two decimal places to the left:

$$\begin{array}{r} 5 \\ \times\, 0.12 \\ \hline 0.60 \end{array}$$

5 — There are no decimal places to the right of this whole number.
×0.12 — There are 2 decimal places in this factor.

The answer must have 2 decimal places. Beginning at the far right, move 2 places to the left and place the decimal.

Practice Set VI – 1

Determine the placement of the decimal point for each of the products shown.

1. $\begin{array}{r} 0.35 \\ \times\ 4 \\ \hline 140 \end{array}$

2. $\begin{array}{r} 94 \\ \times\ 0.4 \\ \hline 376 \end{array}$

3. $\begin{array}{r} 0.707 \\ \times 0.2 \\ \hline 1414 \end{array}$

4. $\begin{array}{r} 1.6 \\ \times\ 40 \\ \hline 640 \end{array}$

5. $\begin{array}{r} 0.0638 \\ \times\ 0.78 \\ \hline 49764 \end{array}$

Note: in number **5** the sum of the decimal points to be counted off is *six*. Yet the product has only five digits. In these cases, insert one or more zeros to the *left* of the product in order to have the required number of decimal places. The answer for (**5**) should be: 0.049764

Practice Set VI – 2

Multiply. Place the decimal point in the correct position in the product.

1. $17.5 \times 6 =$

2. $168 \times 0.321 =$

3. $4.8 \times 0.067 =$

4. $0.56 \times 0.83 =$

5. $63 \times 37.91 =$

6. $0.72 \times 0.095 =$

7. Multiply 0.2279 by 0.029

8. Multiply 6.85 by 81.2

9. $306.693 \times 2.61 =$

10. Find the product of 18.35 and 0.065

11. Wages for 29 hours of work at $ 5.12 per hour are ?

12. Find the cost of 212 bushels of corn at $ 3.08 per bushel.

13. Find the cost of 98 bushels of feed at $5.88 per bushel,

14. How much is 32 quarts of milk at $1.19 a quart?

15. 18 dozen eggs at $ 1.55 per dozen is how much?

Decimal Fractions

In the lab, you may need to multiply by 10 or 100 or 1000. These all represent multiples of ten. There is a short cut to multiplying by multiples of ten. For example, multiply 2.4 by 10, 100, and 1000.

$$2.4 \times 10 = 24$$
$$2.4 \times 100 = 240.0$$
$$2.4 \times 1000 = 2400.0$$

When 2.4 is multiplied by 10, How does the decimal place change in the product?

When multiplying a number by ten, move the decimal of that number one place to the right in the product. When multiplying by 1,000 the decimal point is moved three places to the right in the product.

Practice Set VI – 3

Multiply the following.

1. 3.6×10

2. 5.4×1000

3. 0.47×100

4. 9.61×100

5. 2.45×1000

6. 7.1×10

Division of Decimals

Now we learn how to divide using decimals. Recall that in multiplication the answer, or result is called the product. In division, the answer is called the quotient. The number that is being divided is called the dividend; and the number with which the dividend is divided is called the divisor.

Example:

$$divisor \overline{)dividend}^{quotient} \qquad divisor \longrightarrow 6\overline{)42}^{\,7 \leftarrow quotient}_{\,\leftarrow dividend}$$

Suppose we wanted to divide a whole number by some decimal number. Such as: $0.16\overline{)32}$

The divisor is 0.16 and the dividend is 32. With division, the divisor must always be made into a whole number by moving the decimal place to the right. In this case, the decimal point is moved two places to the right. To complement this procedure, we must also then move the decimal place of the dividend two places to the right as well. Finally, place the decimal point in the quotient, the answer, directly above the new position in the dividend. Like this

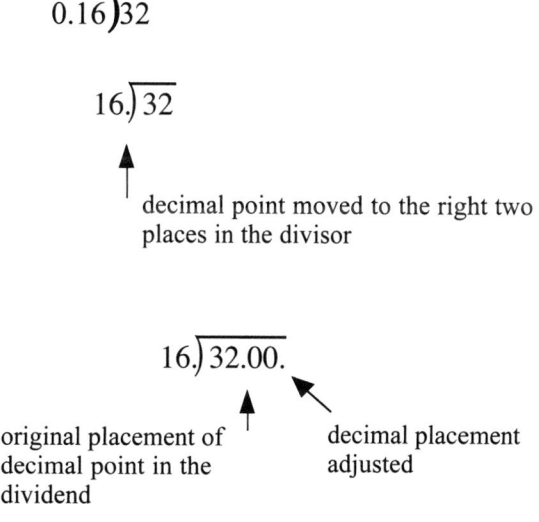

Finally, do the division: $16.\overline{)3200.}^{\,200.}$ The decimal in the quotient is directly above the decimal in the dividend.

Decimal Fractions

Practice Set VI – 4

Divide. Round answer to thousandths (3 places), if necessary.

1. $1.2\overline{)36}$
2. $1.3\overline{)650}$
3. $0.5\overline{)75}$

4. $0.08\overline{)64}$
5. $0.9\overline{)72}$
6. $0.25\overline{)200}$

From (**6**), here is another look at that problem.

$.25\overline{)200}$ = 200 ÷ .25

= 200 ÷ $\frac{1}{4}$ since $0.25 = \frac{1}{4}$

= 200 × $\frac{4}{1}$ as learned when dividing fractions

= 800

To divide a decimal by a whole number, divide as you would for whole numbers and place the decimal point in the quotient directly above the decimal point in the dividend.

Examples:

$16\overline{)6.4}$ = .4 $22\overline{).88}$ = .04 $13\overline{)26.}$ = 2.

Practice Set VI – 5

Divide. Round answers to 3 decimal places, if necessary.

1. $25\overline{)6.50}$
2. $44\overline{)9.24}$
3. $16\overline{).922}$

4. $14\overline{).42}$
5. $12\overline{)2.64}$
6. $25\overline{)1.75}$

7. $25\overline{)75.25}$
8. $47\overline{)317.72}$
9. $64\overline{)131.2}$

To divide a decimal by another decimal, move the decimal point of the divisor to the right until the divisor becomes a whole number. Then move the decimal point in the dividend the same number of places, annexing zeros if necessary. Next, place the decimal point in the quotient. Finally, divide as one would with whole numbers.

Example: 4.5 ÷ 0.15

$$.15\overline{)4.50.} \begin{array}{c}30.\\\end{array}$$

The decimal point in the divisor and the dividend is moved two places to the right.

Practice Set VI – 6

Round answers to three decimal places, if necessary.

1. Divide 9801.9 by 0.9

2. Divide 892.5 by 7.0

3. Divide 58.32 by 1.8

4. Divide 17.28 by 0.12

5. Divide 5.12 by 0.08

6. Divide 3.43 by 0.7

7. Divide 306.72 by 0.8

8. Divide 793.1 by 0.07

9. Divide 100.1 by 0.001

10. Divide 795.07 by 4.3

11. $0.0075 \overline{)0.6}$

12. $0.25 \overline{)75.25}$

13. $4.7 \overline{)317.72}$

14. $6.4 \overline{)873.42}$

Decimal Fractions   73

You have divided decimals into whole numbers, whole numbers into decimals, and decimals into decimals. Now practice placing the decimal point in the quotient.

Practice Set VI – 7

Location of decimal point

The answer for each of the following contains the digits 343. You must correctly place the decimal point in the answer, adding zeros where necessary. The first couple are done for you as examples. It is not necessary to actually do the division since every answer contains the given digits.

1. $124\overline{)42.532}$ = .343

2. $124\overline{)425.32}$ = 3.43

3. $1.24\overline{)42.532}$

4. $.124\overline{)425.32}$

5. $12.4\overline{)4253.2}$

6. $12.4\overline{).42532}$

7. $1.24\overline{)4253.2}$

8. $124\overline{).42532}$

9. $.124\overline{).42532}$

10. $12.4\overline{)4.2532}$

11. $1.24\overline{).042532}$

12. $12.4\overline{)42.532}$

13. $0.124\overline{)4253.2}$

14. $0.124\overline{).042532}$

15. $.00124\overline{).0042532}$

16. $.124\overline{).0042532}$

17. $1.24\overline{).0042532}$

18. $124\overline{).042532}$

74 Decimal Fractions

Practice Set VI – 8 Review

Perform the indicated operation.

1. 0.315
   × 3.12

2. 9.10
   × 9.1

3. 56.7
   × 0.42

4. 0.096
   × 7.8

5. 357.1
   × 0.111

6. 5.03
   × 0.9111

7. 2.56
   × 0.48

8. 600.73
   × 1.12

9. 1.512
   × 1.34

10. 2.432
    × 0.07

11. 0.431
    × 0.32

12. 7.62
    × 3.1

13. 8.031
    × 1.34

14. 1.213
    × 0.561

15. 2.521
    × 6.21

16. 7.36
    × 0.62

17. 9.023
× 1.45

18. 3.123
× 0.654

19. 1.125
× 5.11

20. 6.37
× 0.22

21. 2.5
× 2.1

22. 9.16
× 1.72

23. 15.4
× 1.2

24. 0.0786
× 2.4

25. 14.807
× 4.1

26. 89.7
× 5.3

27. 15.4
× 70

28. 98.23
× 100

29. 14.887
× 0.1

30. 22.73
× 0.01

31. 17.1
× 0.001

32. 12.89
× 0.0001

Divide. Round answers to thousandths, if necessary.

1. $1.8 \div 0.002$

2. $1.616 \div 0.77$

3. $76.4 \div 38.2$

4. $98.65 \div 13.1$

5. $3.6503 \div 1.25$

6. $9.9 \div 3.3$

7. $0.567 \div 14$

8. $3.693 \div 0.03$

9. $50.25 \div 0.5$

10. $200 \div 2.5$

11. $5.40 \div 0.6$

12. $24.57 \div 2.7$

13. $7.5 \div 1.5$

14. $0.006 \div 0.003$

15. $84.84 \div 4.2$

Decimal Fractions

16. $200 \div 2.8$ **17.** $42.63 \div 100$ **18.** $3.655 \div 10$

19. $98.3525 \div 1000$ **20.** $8.359 \div 0.1$ **21.** $8.359 \div 0.01$

22. $8.359 \div 0.001$ **23.** $5.40 \div 0.01$ **24.** $24.56 \div 0.03$

Often, while doing lab work, a need arises to divide by ten, one hundred, 1000, one tenth, one hundredth, or so on. As when multiplying by powers of ten, dividing by powers of ten also can be short cut.

Example: Divide 2.4 by each of the following . . .

$2.4 \div 10 = .24$ $2.4 \div 0.1 = 24$

$2.4 \div 100 = .024$ $2.4 \div 0.01 = 240$

$2.4 \div 1000 = .0024$ $2.4 \div 0.001 = 2400$

In the example above, when we divided 2.4 by 10, how did the decimal point change?

78   Decimal Fractions

You noticed that the decimal point moved one place to the left in the quotient when dividing by ten. When we divided by 0.001 ($^1/_{1000}$) the decimal point moved three places to the *right* in the quotient. So, when dividing by whole number multiples of ten, the decimal point moves one place left in the quotient for each zero in the divisor. In the other direction, division by powers of ten less than one, like $^1/_{10}$ or $^1/_{100}$, the decimal point is adjusted right according to the number of zeros in the divisor.

Practice Set VI – 9

Divide. Practice using the rules for division by powers of 10.

1. $0.01 \overline{)314.2}$

2. $1000 \overline{)314.2}$

3. $10 \overline{)314.2}$

4. $0.001 \overline{)3.142}$

5. $100 \overline{)31.42}$

6. $0.0001 \overline{)314.2}$

7. 314.2 divided *by* 10,000

8. 0.3142 divided by 0.1

9. 100,000 divided *into* 314.2

10. 0.000001 divided into 3.142

Decimal Fractions 79

The following practice set involves multiplying and dividing by powers of ten. This relationship will be further explored with scientific notation later in this chapter. Try using some short cut method when possible.

Practice Set VI – 10 Perform the indicated operation relocating the decimal point as indicated.

Multiply	*Divide*
1. $231 \times 10 =$	$231 \div 10 =$
2. 2001×0.0001	$2001 \div 0.0001$
3. 48.236×1000	$48.236 \div 1000$
4. 2.310×0.01	$2.310 \div 0.01$
5. 4.691×100	$4.691 \div 100$
6. 96.39×1000	$96.39 \div 1000$

7. 856.9 × 0.0001   856.9 ÷ 0.0001

8. 9.8751 × 0.001   9.8751 ÷ 0.001

9. 18.754 × 10   18.754 ÷ 10

10. 910.4 × 100   910.4 ÷ 100

11. 876.12 × 1000   876.12 ÷ 1000

12. 9543.1 × 0.001   9543.1 ÷ 0.001

13. 0.998 × 0.1   0.998 ÷ 0.1

14. 576.24 × 0.0001   576.24 ÷ 0.0001

15. 5.1 × 0.01   5.1 ÷ 0.01

16. 79.99 × 1   79.99 ÷ 1

17. 85.333 × 10000   85.333 ÷ 10000

18. 94.999 × 0.01   94.999 ÷ 0.01

19. 87.632 × 0.001   87.632 ÷ 0.001

20. 994.33 × 0.00001   994.33 ÷ 0.00001

21. 8643.2 × 10   8643.2 ÷ 10

22. 99.999 × 10000   99.999 ÷ 10000

23. 87.432 × 0.001   87.432 ÷ 0.001

24. 8.7432 × 0.01   87.432 ÷ 0.01

Scientific Notation

To convert to scientific notation from a decimal

- based on powers of ten
- Format: $N \times 10^x$ where $1 \leq N < 10$ and x is any integer

Easy to convert by simply moving the decimal point:

- for a number greater than one (1)

⬅ move the decimal point the required "steps" to the Left. The number of steps represents x and x is positive.

- for a number less than 1

➡ move the decimal point the required steps to the Right. The number of steps represents x and x is negative.

Here's how it works ...

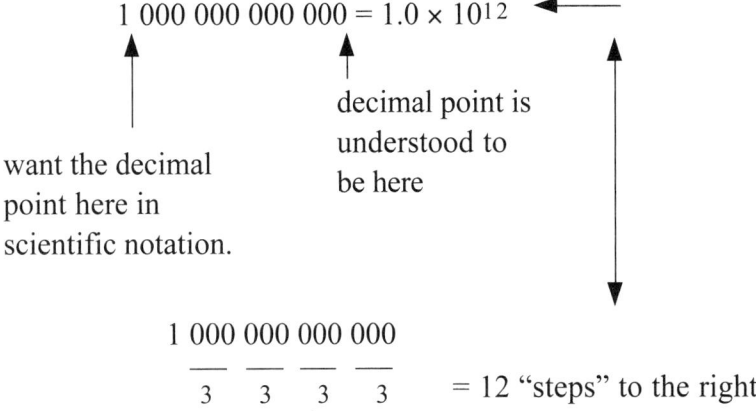

$$1\,000\,000\,000\,000 = 1.0 \times 10^{12}$$

want the decimal point here in scientific notation.

decimal point is understood to be here

$$\underbrace{1\,000}_{3}\,\underbrace{000}_{3}\,\underbrace{000}_{3}\,\underbrace{000}_{3} = 12 \text{ "steps" to the right}$$

... this gives the desired **N** such that **N** is (at least) 1.0 and the power of ten corresponds to the number of places ("steps") taken!

Examples:

$1000 = 1.0 \times 10^3$ $1520 = 1.52 \times 10^3$ $0.003 = 3 \times 10^{-3}$

$0.00415 = 4.15 \times 10^{-3}$ $10004000 = 1.0004 \times 10^7$

$0.0000045 = 4.5 \times 10^{-6}$ $1\,000\,000\,000\,000\,000 = 1.0 \times 10^{15}$

To convert to a decimal from scientific notation

The sign (positive/negative) of the exponent of ten (10^x) determines the direction to move when converting from scientific notation to standard numbers.

- if the sign of the exponent is negative move the decimal that many places left

- if the sign of the exponent is positive, move the decimal point to the right

Examples:

$1.4 \times 10^3 = 1400$ $2.0 \times 10^5 = 200000$ $3.1 \times 10^{-4} = 0.00031$

$9.5 \times 10^{-7} = 0.00000095$ $4.3 \times 10^2 = 430$

$4.5 \times 10^{-6} = 0.0000045$

     move decimal point 6 places to the left (since exponent is *negative*)

You may have noticed that scientific notation with negative exponents indicate decimal numbers less than one. Positive exponents in scientific notation indicate numbers greater than, or equal to, one. Furthermore, any number times one remains the same.

84   Decimal Fractions

Practice Set VI – 11

Express each of the following in scientific notation.

1. 100,000   2. 100   3. 1,000,000

4. 0.0001   5. 0.01   6. 0.00000001

7. 0.0000000001   8. 0.000001   9. 1000

10. 10,000,000

Rewrite each of the following from scientific notation to whole number or decimal notation.

11. 10^6 or 1×10^6 12. 10^4 or 1×10^4 13. 10^3 or 1×10^3

14. 10^7 15. 10^{-3} 16. 10^{-5}

17. 10^{-2} 18. 10^{-6} 19. 10^2

Practice Set VI – 12

Convert to/from scientific notation, as appropriate.

1. 2×10^4 2. 8.4×10^6

3. 0.33×10^{-2} 4. 0.33×10^2

5. 8.47×10^{-8}

6. 0.00035

7. 0.000839

8. 10857

9. 87.69×10^{8}

10. 4.235×10^{-4}

11. 6.798×10^{-7}

12. 246810

13. 0.00357

14. 8.276×10^{-5}

15. 7.5×10^{-6}

16. 15×10^{-6}

17. 4×10^{7}

18. 0.0000436

19. 45789

20. 257

21. 8324.67

22. 2.69×10^4

23. 0.00357

24. 0.00005

25. 0.00001

Fraction Review

Add and reduce to lowest terms.

1. $2\frac{2}{9}$
   $1\frac{1}{27}$
   $\frac{6}{18}$
   $+\frac{1}{3}$

2. $5\frac{1}{8}$
   $2\frac{3}{64}$
   $\frac{5}{24}$
   $+3\frac{1}{4}$

3. $6\frac{1}{4}$
   $\frac{5}{6}$
   $12\frac{5}{8}$
   $+\frac{12}{32}$

4. $5\frac{6}{8}$
   $6\frac{1}{4}$
   $12\frac{1}{6}$
   $+1\frac{3}{8}$

5. $\frac{7}{8}$
   $\frac{3}{4}$
   $+\frac{9}{10}$

Convert to mixed or whole numbers. Reduce and express in lowest terms.

6. $\frac{20}{5} =$

7. $\frac{16}{5} =$

8. $\frac{50}{6} =$

9. $\frac{13}{12} =$

10. $\frac{36}{12} =$

11. $\frac{56}{6} =$

12. $\frac{42}{3} =$

13. $\frac{19}{4} =$

14. $\frac{72}{8} =$

15. $\frac{7}{2} =$

88 Fraction Review

Multiply. Reduce to lowest terms.

16. $\dfrac{2}{3} \times \dfrac{5}{12} =$

17. $1\dfrac{1}{4} \times 5\dfrac{1}{8} =$

18. $2\dfrac{1}{2} \times 3\dfrac{2}{3} \times 4\dfrac{5}{8} =$

19. $\dfrac{7}{9} \times \dfrac{1}{5} =$

20. $2\dfrac{3}{5} \times 4\dfrac{1}{5} =$

21. $\dfrac{24}{25} \times \dfrac{11}{20} =$

22. $1\dfrac{3}{4} \times 2\dfrac{3}{4} =$

23. $3\dfrac{3}{4} \times 1\dfrac{3}{5} \times 2\dfrac{4}{5} =$

24. $\dfrac{1}{3} \times 4\dfrac{1}{2} =$

25. $\dfrac{5}{12} \times \dfrac{2}{3} =$

26. $3\dfrac{1}{6} \times 3\dfrac{1}{4} =$

27. $\dfrac{3}{4} \times \dfrac{2}{5} =$

28. $6\dfrac{1}{2} \times 4\dfrac{7}{8} =$

29. $\dfrac{3}{5} \times \dfrac{3}{2} =$

30. $8\dfrac{2}{5} \times 2\dfrac{3}{5} =$

31. $\dfrac{5}{8} \times \dfrac{4}{5} =$

32. $2\dfrac{1}{3} \times 4\dfrac{5}{12} =$

33. $12\dfrac{1}{2} \times 17\dfrac{1}{3} \times 3\dfrac{3}{4} =$

Subtract and reduce to lowest terms.

34. $\dfrac{7}{8}$
$-\dfrac{1}{4}$

35. $5\dfrac{4}{5}$
$-2\dfrac{3}{5}$

36. $12\dfrac{1}{2}$
$-2\dfrac{1}{6}$

37. $\dfrac{9}{10}$
$-\dfrac{3}{5}$

38. $15\dfrac{2}{3}$
$-3\dfrac{2}{3}$

39. $\dfrac{7}{10}$
$-\dfrac{2}{5}$

40. $\dfrac{11}{16}$
$-\dfrac{1}{2}$

41. $19\dfrac{1}{2}$
$-11\dfrac{1}{4}$

42. $61\dfrac{2}{3}$
$-2\dfrac{4}{5}$

43. $1\dfrac{1}{2}$
$-\dfrac{3}{4}$

Fraction Review

Divide. Reduce to lowest terms.

44. $8\dfrac{5}{8} \div \dfrac{1}{50} =$

45. $\dfrac{4}{75} \div \dfrac{7}{25} =$

46. $12\dfrac{4}{5} \div 5\dfrac{1}{2} =$

47. $25\dfrac{1}{2} \div 7\dfrac{3}{4} =$

48. $\dfrac{3}{20} \div \dfrac{1}{2} =$

49. $\dfrac{4}{25} \div \dfrac{8}{25} =$

50. $190\dfrac{3}{4} \div 2\dfrac{5}{8} =$

51. $4\dfrac{1}{5} \div 2\dfrac{9}{10} =$

52. $1\dfrac{1}{2} \div \dfrac{3}{4} =$

Unit II

Chapter 7
Percentage

There is a need to know how to compute percentage both in business and industry. Many handbooks, manuals, and catalogs make references to percents. The sign, or symbol, for percent is %. Percent means *per hundred.* Per means divide, and cent refers to 100. Thus, percent means something divided by 100. 40% is read forty percent and indicates 40 hundredths or 40 parts out of 100.

Changing Percent to a Number

Math operations involving percentages, such as multiplication and division, cannot be computed in the form using the symbol %. We must change the percent into a decimal or common fraction. Since percent means hundredths, we can change percent into a decimal. Recall that hundred*ths* is two (decimal) places to the right of the decimal point. In a whole number, the decimal is understood to be at the rightmost place of the number.

Examples: 8 is the same as 8.0
97 is the same as 97.0

When multiplying a number by 100, we learned to move the decimal point two places to the right. If dividing by 100, move the decimal two places to the left. Percent means divide by 100. Therefore, to change a percent to a decimal drop the % sign and move the decimal two places to the left.

Examples: 81% = 0.81
96% = 0.96
5% = 0.05
112% = 1.12

Percentage

Practice Set VII – 1

Change the following % to decimals.

1. 15%   2. 1%   3. 94.3%

4. 33%   5. 9%   6. 100%

7. 40%   8. 125%   9. 5%

To change a decimal to a percent move the decimal point two places to the right and append the percent sign, %.

Examples: 0.12 = 12%

0.07 = 7%

1.19 = 119%

Practice Set VII – 2

Change the following decimals to percent:

1. 0.10   2. 6.3   3. 0.9

4. 0.12   5. 0.762   6. .375

7. 0.125   8. 0.875   9. .085

10. 0.09   11. 2.25   12. 0.1

Percentage

To change from a percent to a common fraction requires expressing the value of the percent as a fraction rather than a decimal. To do this, use the value of the percent as the numerator and 100 as the denominator. Reduce as necessary.

Examples: $21\% = \dfrac{21}{100}$ $\qquad 40\% = \dfrac{40}{100} = \dfrac{2}{5}$ $\qquad 75\% = \dfrac{75}{100} = \dfrac{3}{4}$

Practice Set VII – 3

Change the given percents to common fractions. Be sure to reduce.

1. 60%   2. 10%   3. 110%

4. 50%   5. 8%   6. 90%

To change any fraction to percent, first change the fraction to a decimal by dividing the denominator into the numerator. Then change the resulting decimal to a percent as previously discussed. *(See Practice Set VII – 2.)*

Examples: Change $\dfrac{1}{2}$ to percent $\qquad 2\overline{)1.0} = 0.5 = 50\%$

Write $3/8$ as a percent $\qquad \dfrac{3}{8} = 8\overline{)3.000} = 0.375 = 37.5\%$

Practice Set VII – 4

Change the following fractions to percents. If necessary, round to the nearest tenth of a percent

1. $\dfrac{1}{4}$

2. $\dfrac{1}{12}$

3. $\dfrac{5}{6}$

4. $\dfrac{3}{5}$

5. $\dfrac{3}{16}$

6. $\dfrac{1}{5}$

7. $\dfrac{7}{10}$

8. $\dfrac{7}{8}$

Practice Set VII – 5

Express each of the following percents as a decimal.

1. 12.5%

2. 8.5%

3. 57.11%

4. 6.25%

5. 9.5%

6. 190%

Express each of the following decimals as a percent.

7. 0.33 **8.** 0.3633 **9.** 0.987

10. 0.63 **11.** 0.11 **12.** 16.375

Express each of the following fractions to the nearest tenth of a percent.

13. $\dfrac{1}{8}$ **14.** $\dfrac{5}{8}$ **15.** $\dfrac{1}{7}$

16. $\dfrac{4}{7}$ **17.** $\dfrac{1}{9}$ **18.** $\dfrac{5}{9}$

19. $\dfrac{1}{11}$ **20.** $\dfrac{7}{11}$

Express each of the following percents as a common fraction and reduce to lowest terms where necessary.

Examples: $5\% = \dfrac{5}{100} = \dfrac{1}{20}$ Or, working with the decimal form $5\% = .05 = \dfrac{5}{100} = \dfrac{1}{20}$

$$12.5\% = .125 = \dfrac{125}{1000} = \dfrac{1}{8}$$

21. 2%   **22.** 72%   **23.** 20%

24. 40%   **25.** 32%   **26.** 48%

27. 38.5%   **28.** 1.75%

Complete the following chart. Express each of the following as a percent, as a decimal and/or a fraction or mixed number.

	Fraction	Decimal	Percent
29.			8%
30.			7.5%
31.		0.925	
32.			66.7%
33.	$\dfrac{3}{7}$		
34.		0.125	
35.		650.00	
36.	$\dfrac{9}{16}$		
37.			125%
38.	$\dfrac{11}{42}$		
39.		0.333	
40.	$3\dfrac{5}{8}$		
41.	$1\dfrac{5}{9}$		
42.			3.25%

Percentage

Now that we know the mechanics of changing percents to decimals and fractions and back again, we can use that knowledge to solve problems involving percentages. To find the percent of a given number use the following guidelines:

- Convert the percent to either a fractional or decimal equivalent.
- Multiply the given number by this equivalent.
- Label answer with appropriate unit of measure.

Example: (i) Find 16% of 1218 millimeters.

Step 1: Change 16% to a decimal   16% = .16

Step 2: Multiply

```
  1218
  x.16
 ─────
 194.88
```

Step 3: Label answer   194.88 millimeters is 16% of 1218 ml

(ii) Follow the same steps when the percent is a mixed number.

Find $6 \tfrac{1}{4}$ % of 782 hours

Step 1: $6 \tfrac{1}{4}$ % = 6.25% = 0.0625

Step 2:
```
        782
      x.0625
      48.8750
```

Step 3: 48.875 hours

Here is one way to think about percentage problems. Consider –

x percent   of   **n**   is   **y**

Of means "times" and *is* means "equals". *x percent* must be a decimal to perform any arithmetic. *n* generally is the total, or original amount. *y* is the part of the total, or the amount of increase, or the amount of decrease. You will always know, or be able to determine, two of these three parts.

A way to remember this is to make a sentence as a mnemonic device. For example, "What percent of something is this?"

Percentage

	$x\%$	of	n	is	y	

What percent of something is this?

① × ② = ③

(1) 35% of 52 is ?
In this case, the model is   35% × 52 = ???   change 35% to a decimal and multiply (= 18.2)

(2) What percent of 52 is 18.2?   ??? × 52 = 18.2   divide 18.2 by 52; change the resultant decimal to percent (.35 = 35%)

(3) 35% of what is 18.2?   35% × ??? = 18.2   divide 18.2 by 0.35 to get 52

Practice Set VII – 6

Solve each of the following. Round answer to three places, if necessary.

1. 5% of 1000

2. 20% of 555

3. 50% of 1000

4. 12.5% of 480

5. 6.25% of 800

6. 33.3% of 500

7. 10% of 750

8. 20% of 500

9. 25% of 1200

10. 37.5% of 1200

11. 16.67% of 180

12. 40% of 1200

Word problems are practical situations where various mathematical procedures are used. The following is an example of percentage word problems.

Example:

A clinic has 43,560 square feet of floor space. An expansion is planned that will increase the floor space 25%. (a) Find the amount of floor space that is being added. (b) Find the total floor space after the addition.

$$\begin{array}{r} 43,560 \\ \times\, 0.25 \\ \hline 10,890.00 \end{array}$$ (a) 25% of 43,560 is added floor space: 10,890 sq. ft.

(b) 43,560 sq. ft. + 10,890 sq. ft. = 54,450 sq. ft.
floor space + increased space = total floor space after addition

Practice Set VII – 7

Solve the following word problems. Round to two places, if necessary.

1. One veterinarian figured a procedure at a cost of $940.00. A second doctor quoted a price that was 25% less. What was the second price?

2. Seventy-five pounds of brass contains 45% zinc and the balance is copper. Determine the number of pounds of zinc.

3. A shipment of chemicals was billed at $548.00 but it was damaged in transit. An allowance of 15% was made for the damages. What is the net amount due?

4. A technician measured 500 ml of distilled water. Eighteen percent of the water was used in the lab. How much distilled water was left?

Determining what percent one number is of another

Example: 20 is what percent of 50   or written another way: 20 = ? % of 50

   y is x %   of n

Write the numbers as a fraction. The number to be compared (20) is the numerator. The number with which it to be compared (50) is the denominator.

$$\text{Part} \rightarrow \frac{20}{50} = \frac{2}{5}$$
$$\text{Total, or original} \rightarrow$$

change the fraction to a decimal

$$5\overline{)2.0} = .4$$

change 0.4 to percent

$$0.4 = 40\% \quad 20 \text{ is } 40\% \text{ of } 50.$$

20 is the part of the total 50. Divide the part by the total or original amount.

Example: In measuring 80 lbs. of chemicals, 1.6 pounds was lost by accident. What percent was lost?

1.6 = ? % of 80   Thus, $\text{Part} \rightarrow \frac{1.6}{80}$
                          $\text{Total, or original} \rightarrow$

Simplifying $80\overline{)1.60} = .02$ writing the decimal as a percent   0.02 = 2% was lost

Practice Set VII – 8

Solve the following problems. Round percents to nearest tenth percent. Round decimal answers to two decimal places.

1. 27 lbs. of lab chemicals were ordered, but 8 lbs. were lost in shipment. What percent was lost?

2. Given 125 lbs. of chemicals, 2.56 lbs. was lost. What percent was lost?

3. The lab had 11 lbs. of chemicals, 1.1 lbs. were lost. What percent loss is this?

4. Inspecting 50 bottles used for dispensing medication, 4 were found to be broken. What percent were broken?

5. In working 45 problems on a test, 7 were incorrect. What percent were incorrect?

6. After 11 days at work you missed a day. What percent of those 12 days total have you missed?

7. A man working for $6.40 per hour has his pay increased by 52 cents per hour. What percent increase did he receive?

8. John feeds his dogs 2 3/4 pounds of dog food from a canister containing 12 lbs. of food. What percent of the food is removed for each feeding?

9. For a certain laboratory experiment, a resultant weighing 3.25 lbs. is obtained. If the total weight of the chemical components of the experiment were 4.59 lbs. , then the weight of the resultant is what percent of the components?

10. Raw materials for a certain type of animal cage weigh 327 lbs. A finished cage weighs 288 lbs. What percent of the raw material is lost in manufacture?

Percentage

Determining a new price when there is a percent change is common. This could be the result of a price increase due to inflation or a price decrease due to a discount. Either way, the procedures are similar.

Price Increase

1. Find the change by converting the percent to its decimal equivalent and multiplying by the price.
2. Add the increase in the price to the original price to find the new price.

Example: 9% increase in an object which originally cost $15.49

$$9\% = 0.09 \quad \text{Use the decimal equivalent}$$

$x\%$ of n is y

9% of 15.49 is

$0.09 \cdot 15.49 =$

$15.49		$15.49	Original cost
$\times 0.09$	Compute the price increase	+ 1.39	Amount of increase
$1.3941 = $1.39		$16.88	Total new price

Price Decrease

1. Find the change by converting the percent to its decimal equivalent and multiplying by the price.
2. Subtract the decrease in price from the original price to find the new price.

Example: 6% decrease in cost of an object which originally cost $8.95

$$6\% = 0.06 \quad \text{Use the decimal equivalent}$$

6% of 8.95 is

$$0.06 \cdot 8.95 =$$

$8.95	Original cost	$8.95	Original price
× 0.06	Amount of decrease	− 0.54	Price decrease
$0.537 = $0.54		$8.41	Total new price

Practice Set VII – 9

Find the new cost for each of the following.

1. 6.6% increase on an original price of $5.47

2. 5% decrease on an original price of $10.

3. 2% decrease from an original price of $5.39

4. 8% increase from an original price of $3.35

5. 11% increase on an original price of $6.98

Practice Set VII – 10

Evaluate each of the following. Round answer to 2 places, if needed.

1. 16% of 28

2. 90% of 1,000

3. 10% of 1,600

4. 17% of 32

5. 11 1/2% of 980

6. 13% of 78

7. 1/4% of 13

8. 7 1/4% of 100

9. The kennel area is to be enlarged by 25%. The present size is 1,230 square feet. **a**. How much additional space will be available? **b**. What will be the total area when complete?

Practice Set VII – 11

The following items are taken from two price lists. Company A gives a 22% discount, while Company B's prices have increased by 7 1/2%. Find the new prices of each company.

Item	Company A list price	Company A new price	Company B list price	Company B new price
general operating scissors	$6.10		$4.45	
Metzenbaum scissors	$8.30		$6.25	
iris scissors	$7.05		$5.00	
Allis tissue forceps	$7.58		$5.55	
surgical cotton wadding	$4.20		$3.85	
Kelly forceps	$5.20		$3.52	
Needle holders	$4.25		$3.00	
Gauze sponges	$60.00/cs		$42.75/cs	
Endotracheal tubes	$2.38		$1.93	
First-aid dressing	$15/dz.		$14.50/dz.	
Mayo intestinal needles	$9.20/dz.		$8.75/dz.	

Solutions – General

The term *grams per deciliter* is used in hospital medicine. For example, determining the amount of hemoglobin in the blood is expressed as 14 g/dl, which means the number of grams per 100 ml or grams per deciliter. *Gram percent* (g%) means grams per 100 ml. Both grams percent for grams per 100 ml and grams per deciliter are terms used. However, the term gram per deciliter has become popular in recent times.

Example: 12 grams in 100 ml. of solution is termed 12 gram percent or 12 g% or 12 g/dl.

Note that 100 ml = 1 deciliter $\quad \dfrac{12\,g}{100\,ml} = \dfrac{12\,g}{1\,dl}$

Practice Set VII – 12

Express each of the following as grams percent or grams per 100 ml.

1. 14 g/100 ml =

2. 0.9 g/100 ml =

3. 0.5 g/100 ml =

4. 1 g/100 ml =

5. 4 g/100 ml =

Sometimes the quantity is very small and the term milligram percent (mg%) is used. This means the number of mg per 100 ml or the number of mg per deciliter.

Example: 5 mg in 100 ml of solution is termed 5 mg percent or 5 mg%

Convert:

  6. 3.2 mg/100 ml =   **7.** 0.4 mg/100 ml =

Practice Set VII – 13

The *packed cell volume* (PCV) in blood analysis is divided by 3 to obtain the amount of hemoglobin (Hb) in the blood. This is recorded in g/100 ml or gram percent or gram/deciliter. Calculate the following in g% (The weight of Hb is measured in grams and the volume of blood in ml.)

Example: PCV was measured at 51. $51 \div 3 = 17$ so Hb is 17g% or 17 g/dl

	PCV	
1.	36	dog_1
2.	22	dog_2
3.	24	cat_1
4.	42	cat_2
5.	30	pig_1
6.	48	pig_2

Percentage

Solutions whose concentration are given in % means the number of grams (g) of a substance per 100 milliliters (ml) of solution or, if liquid, the number of milliliters of a substance per 100 milliliters of the solution. Calculate the concentration in % for each of the following.

Examples: (i) 12.5 g of sodium chloride in 100 ml of solution would be a 12.5% solution of sodium chloride. (ii) 22 ml of Formalin (a liquid chemical) in 100 ml of solution would be a 22% solution of Formalin.

7. 0.9 g of sodium chloride in 100 ml of solution

8. 5 g of dextrose in 100 ml of solution

9. 4.5 g of dextrose in 100 ml of solution

10. 10 ml of formalin in 100 ml of solution

11. 2 g of copper sulfate in 100 ml of solution

12. 1 g of copper sulfate in 100 ml of solution

13. 70 ml of isopropyl alcohol in 100 ml of solution

14. 2 ml of formalin in 100 ml of solution

Chapter 8
Ratio and Proportion

The study of ratios provides the background necessary to solve dosage problems involving ratio and proportion.

The comparison of one quantity with another like quantity is called a ratio. For example, suppose you compare a dime and a nickel. Both involve money, but are of different size and weight (among other differences.) We could compare their values and write a ratio as 10 cents to 5 cents. We could indicate this ratio as 10 : 5 using a colon to represent the ratio 10 to 5. Another way this ratio could be represented is as a fraction: $\frac{10}{5}$.

All the rules governing fractions apply to ratios as well.

Example:
Compare these two circles:

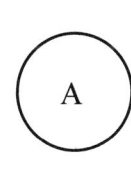
Diameter: 9

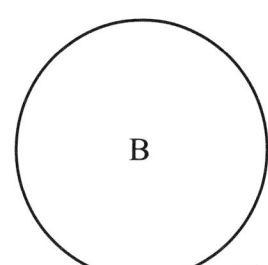
Diameter: 15

The diameter of circle A compared to the diameter of circle B may be written as the *ratio*:

$$9 \text{ to } 15 \quad \text{or} \quad 9:15 \quad \text{or} \quad \frac{9}{15}$$

This last can be reduced: $\frac{9}{15} = \frac{3}{5}$ $\frac{3}{5}$ or 3 : 5

Ratios are always expressed in lowest terms (as are fractions).

Examples: (i) 5:10 or $\frac{5}{10} = \frac{1}{2}$ or 1 : 2

(ii) 3:9 or $\frac{3}{9} = \frac{1}{3}$ or 1 : 3

Ratio and Proportion

Practice Set VIII – 1

Read the following problems and express the information given as a ratio.

1. If graduated cylinder "A" has 80 milliliters of solution and a second graduated cylinder "B" has 40 milliliters of the solution, what is the ratio of "A" to "B"?   [80:40 = 2:1]

2. Refer to the previous problem (a). What is the ratio of "B" to "A"?

3. Two dogs, "A" and "B" are weighed separately. "A" weighs 60 pounds and "B" weighs 25 pounds. What is the (weight) ratio of "A" to "B"?

4. a. A solution mixture has the ratio of one part hydrochloric acid (HCL), 70 parts Ethyl Alcohol (EtOH), and 29 parts water. What is the ratio of EtOH to water?

b. In the part **a** of this problem, what is the ratio of water to HCL?

The *value* of a ratio is found by dividing the numerator by the denominator to make a decimal number.

Examples:

(i) 4:5 or $\frac{4}{5}$ $\longrightarrow$ $\frac{4}{5} = 0.8$

(ii) 3:6 or $\frac{3}{6}$ $\longrightarrow$ $\frac{3}{6} = \frac{1}{2} = 0.5$

Ratio and Proportion 117

Examples: (i) 4 : 32 $\dfrac{4}{32} = \dfrac{1}{8} = 0.125$

(ii) 6 : 18 $6/18 = 1/3 = 0.33$ [Note the value of 6:18 is equal to the value of 1:3]

Practice Set VIII – 2

Convert each ratio to fraction form (reduce where necessary) and find the value of the ratio to nearest hundredth.

1. 5 : 15
2. 9 : 81
3. 17 : 51

4. 6 : 12
5. 8 : 64
6. 9 : 10

Ratios usually have the same units.

Examples: (i) 10 feet : 40 feet   (ii) 1 cc : 50 cc   (iii) 4 in : 40 in

However, in clinical laboratory conditions, ratios *may* have dissimilar units. Ratios with dissimilar units are called *rates*. We can reduce ratios without affecting the units.

Examples: (i) 5 mg : 1 cc   (ii) 1 cc : 5 lb. body wt.

$\dfrac{5mg}{1cc}$ $\dfrac{1cc}{5lbs}$

(iii) 15 g : 100 ml = $\dfrac{15\,g}{100\,ml} = \dfrac{3\,g}{20\,ml}$

Practice Set VIII – 3

Write the ratios for the following. Be sure to include units.

1. There are 5 grams of Surital found in 100 ml of a saline solution.

2. 10 mg of sodium caparsolate are dissolved in 1 ml of solution.

3. There are 100 mg of Thiamin in every 1 cc of solution.

4. The dosage for Vitamin B complex is 1 cc for every 100 lbs. body weight.

5. Thorazine contains 25 mg in every ml in liquid form.

6. 0.1 mg of Thorazine is given for every 2.0 kg of body weight.

7. 1 cc of sodium pentobarbital is given for every 5 lb of body weight.

Ratio and Proportion   119

Medicine bottles and labels

Working in a clinic or lab may involve using the information from a medicine bottle label or package insert to determine dosage. It is your responsibility to determine the correct dosage for the patient even if the unit dosage is provided.

A lot of information is provided on the medicine bottle label itself and / or the package insert. Your understanding and comprehension of dosage and concentration and their meanings cannot be minimized.

You may be given the opportunity to learn and practice reading and interpreting the dosage and concentration information commonly found on a label.

Dosage is the rate of administration, generally provided in terms of how much to administer per pound, kilogram, or individual animal type.

Examples: 5 mg per 10 lbs or $\dfrac{5mg}{10lbs}$

1 cc per 5 lbs body weight or $\dfrac{1cc}{5lbs}$

1 capsule per individual

1 cc per 1 kg or $\dfrac{1cc}{1kg}$

Concentration is expressed in terms of how much active ingredient per unit of medication.

Examples: $\dfrac{5\ mg}{\text{tablet}}$ $\dfrac{250\ mg}{\text{capsule}}$ $\dfrac{1000\ mg}{1\ \text{cc}}$

Ratio and Proportion

Most dosage problems can be solved using proportions. A *proportion* is composed of two ratios that are equal. The ratios 1 : 2 and 12 : 24 form a proportion since the two ratios are equal. A proportion can be written 1 : 2 = 12 : 24 which is read " 1 is to 2 as 12 is to 24." A proportion is more commonly written as $\frac{1}{2} = \frac{12}{24}$. Typically, three of the values are known and there is an unknown fourth value. You can determine the unknown value by using a technique called cross–multiplication to solve the proportion.

The parts of a proportion: If we had two ratios such as 1 : 3 and 4 : 12 which represent equal quantities, one way they can be expressed as a proportion is …

$$\underset{\text{means}}{\overset{\text{extremes}}{1 : 3 = 4 : 12}}$$

The two outside terms of a proportion (1 and 12) are called extremes. The two inner terms (3 and 4) are called means. In any proportion, the product of the extremes equals the product of the means. $1 \times 12 = 3 \times 4$

The most common method to express a proportion is in fraction form.

Example: 1 : 3 = 4 : 12   can be written $\frac{1}{3} = \frac{4}{12}$

When written in this manner, a missing, or unknown, element of the proportion can be determined by cross-multiplying.

Example: 2 : 5 = 8 : n   or $\frac{2}{5} = \frac{8}{n}$ n represents the unknown term

   cross-multiply: 2 x n = 2n   and 5 x 8 = 40

   yields the equation: 2n = 40

In order to solve this equation, the 2 must be eliminated from the left–hand side of the equation. Since 2n indicates multiplication, undo that by using division. Divide each side of the equation by 2.

$$\frac{2n}{2} = \frac{40}{2}$$ dividing both sides of the equation by 2 and canceling the twos on the left-hand side

$$n = 20$$

Check for the correct solution by multiplying the means and the extremes: $2 \times 20 = 5 \times 8$!

Some helpful rules governing proportions:

Both sides of the proportion equality can be:

- multiplied by the same number without changing the value of the proportion.
- divided by the same number without changing the value of the proportion.
- added to by the same number without changing the value of the proportion.
- subtracted to or from by the same number without changing its value.
- inverted without changing its value.

Tip: to solve a proportion by cross-multiplication, multiply the two numbers diagonally opposite each other and divide by the number that is diagonally opposite the unknown.

Examples: (i)

$$\frac{12}{3} = \frac{n}{4}$$

multiply the two numbers diagonally opposite

divide this product by the number diagonally opposite the unknown (here it's 3)

$$n = (12 \times 4) \div 3$$

$$n = 48 \div 3$$

$$n = 16$$

122   Ratio and Proportion

(ii) $\dfrac{n}{7} \diagup \dfrac{10}{35}$ multiply diagonally across the equals sign; divide by the 35 since 35 has no number to multiply by

$n = \dfrac{7 \times 10}{35}$

$n = 2$

(iii) $\dfrac{5}{n} = \dfrac{35}{56}$

$n = \dfrac{5 \times 56}{35}$

$n = 8$

Note that cancellation techniques **cannot** be used across equals signs.

Practice Set VIII – 4

Find the value of the unknown term in each of the following proportions. Round to nearest hundredth.

1. $n : 200 = 1 : 10$

2. $1 : 15 = 0.2 : n$

3. $1 : 15 = 0.1 : x$

(Notice the complex fraction in #5.)

4. $\dfrac{x}{2000} = \dfrac{.85}{100}$

5. $\dfrac{\frac{1}{6}}{\frac{1}{8}} = \dfrac{x}{30}$

6. $\dfrac{3}{6} = \dfrac{1}{x}$

7. $\dfrac{1}{5000} = \dfrac{.2}{a}$

8. $\dfrac{2}{n} = \dfrac{22}{33}$

9. $\dfrac{0.9}{100} = \dfrac{x}{1000}$

10. $\dfrac{14}{n} = \dfrac{7}{28}$

11. $\dfrac{10}{100} = \dfrac{x}{4}$

12. $\dfrac{x}{16} = \dfrac{8}{64}$

13. $5:100 = 20:x$

14. $\dfrac{14}{12} = \dfrac{7}{x}$

15. $\dfrac{1}{50} = \dfrac{x}{\frac{1}{2}}$

16. If 9 dogs cages cost $450, how many cages can be purchased for $1000 ?

17. If 8 dog feeders cost $72, how much will 19 dog feeders cost?

18. The number of WBC (white blood cells) can be estimated using viscosity measurements. Assuming a linear relationship, what is the estimated WBC count when the average flow time is 5 seconds if a 5000 WBC has an average flow time of 6 seconds?

Problems found in a clinical setting usually have units associated with them. When solving these problems, make certain to include the units. Units, by the way, will "cancel" just as numbers did when multiplying and dividing fractions and the same rules apply.

124   Ratio and Proportion

Note: since the letter "x" is frequently used to signify, or stand in for, an unknown quantity, we will use the more conventional "dot (•) or an asterisk (*)" to signify multiplication.

Example: $\dfrac{x}{5lbs} = \dfrac{2mg}{10lbs}$ cross-multiply as usual

$x = \dfrac{2mg \cdot 5lbs}{10lbs}$ the pounds units cancel

$x = \dfrac{2mg \cdot \overset{1}{\cancel{5}}}{\underset{2}{\cancel{10}}}$ cancel numbers if possible

$x = \dfrac{2mg}{2}$ continue canceling; remember $\dfrac{2}{2} = 1$

$x = 1mg$

The units can also be used to check the result. If the answer had been in pounds, there would have been some type of error somewhere. A useful procedure is to make sure the units in the two numerators match each other and the units in the two denominators also match one another.

Practice Set VIII – 5

Solve the following proportions. Be sure your answer includes the proper units.

1. $\dfrac{300mg}{x} = \dfrac{10mg}{1ml}$

2. $\dfrac{2lbs}{4cc} = \dfrac{10lbs}{x}$

3. $\dfrac{x}{10lbs} = \dfrac{1cc}{25lbs}$

4. $\dfrac{x}{1400lbs} = \dfrac{5mg}{100lbs}$

Chapter 8 Review

Solve each of the following. Be sure to show units where applicable. Round answers to 3 decimal places when necessary.

1. $\dfrac{x}{2} = \dfrac{3}{6}$

2. $\dfrac{x}{8} = \dfrac{10}{16}$

3. $\dfrac{x}{17} = \dfrac{3}{51}$

4. $\dfrac{x}{9} = \dfrac{21}{24}$

5. $\dfrac{x}{6} = \dfrac{3}{16}$

6. $\dfrac{x}{7} = \dfrac{5}{9}$

7. $\dfrac{x}{3} = \dfrac{9}{1}$

8. $\dfrac{x}{2.5} = \dfrac{8}{3}$

9. $\dfrac{8}{x} = \dfrac{16}{3}$

10. $\dfrac{4}{x} = \dfrac{7}{11}$

11. $\dfrac{3}{4} = \dfrac{75}{x}$

12. $\dfrac{2.5}{6} = \dfrac{x}{25}$

13. $\dfrac{13}{14} = \dfrac{10}{x}$

14. $\dfrac{12}{30} = \dfrac{x}{5}$

15. $\dfrac{13}{39} = \dfrac{9}{x}$

16. $\dfrac{14}{28} = \dfrac{x}{8.5}$

17. $\dfrac{3}{9} = \dfrac{5}{x}$

18. $\dfrac{1.8mg}{1cc} = \dfrac{3.5mg}{x}$

19. $\dfrac{1cc}{5lbs} = \dfrac{x}{35lbs}$

20. $\dfrac{1cc}{10lbs} = \dfrac{x}{35lbs}$

21. $\dfrac{1cc}{5lbs} = \dfrac{x}{65lbs}$

22. $\dfrac{x}{7.5lbs} = \dfrac{0.25mg}{1lb}$

23. $\dfrac{1drop}{5cc} = \dfrac{n}{35cc}$

24. $\dfrac{10mg}{1ml} = \dfrac{70mg}{x}$

25. $\dfrac{55mg}{n} = \dfrac{10mg}{1ml}$

26. $\dfrac{0.5mg}{1cc} = \dfrac{7.5mg}{a}$

27. $\dfrac{1cc}{25lbs} = \dfrac{a}{58lbs}$

28. $\dfrac{x}{500ml} = \dfrac{4g}{100ml}$

29. $\dfrac{a}{1000ml} = \dfrac{0.9g}{100ml}$

30. $\dfrac{160mg}{n} = \dfrac{40mg}{1cc}$

31. $\dfrac{x}{17lbs} = \dfrac{1mg}{1lb}$

32. $\dfrac{x}{30cc} = \dfrac{1drop}{5cc}$

33. $\dfrac{x}{5.5lbs} = \dfrac{0.5mg}{1lb}$

34. $\dfrac{x}{5.5lbs} = \dfrac{0.25mg}{1lb}$

35. $\dfrac{x}{800ml} = \dfrac{2.5g}{100ml}$

36. $\dfrac{160mg}{x} = \dfrac{20mg}{1cc}$

37. $\dfrac{180mg}{x} = \dfrac{6mg}{10cc}$

38. $\dfrac{x}{25lbs} = \dfrac{\frac{1}{4}mg}{1lb}$

39. $\dfrac{x}{24cc} = \dfrac{1drop}{5cc}$

40. $\dfrac{325mg}{x} = \dfrac{25mg}{1ml}$

41. $\dfrac{x}{14lb} = \dfrac{0.25mg}{1lb}$

42. $\dfrac{20mg}{1cc} = \dfrac{3.50mg}{x}$

43. $\dfrac{x}{1600 lbs} = \dfrac{2mg}{100 lbs}$

44. $\dfrac{32mg}{x} = \dfrac{10mg}{1ml}$

45. $\dfrac{x}{1250 lbs} = \dfrac{4mg}{100 lbs}$

46. $\dfrac{x}{2000 lbs} = \dfrac{3mg}{100 lbs}$

47. $\dfrac{n}{25 lbs} = \dfrac{1cc}{5 lbs}$

48. $\dfrac{5mg}{n} = \dfrac{6mg}{1ml}$

49. $\dfrac{13mg}{x} = \dfrac{25mg}{1ml}$

50. $\dfrac{n}{7.5 lbs} = \dfrac{0.1mg}{1lb}$

51. $\dfrac{18mg}{x} = \dfrac{20mg}{1ml}$

52. $\dfrac{0.5mg}{1lb} = \dfrac{x}{8.5 lbs}$

53. $\dfrac{x}{9 lbs} = \dfrac{1cc}{25 lbs}$

54. $\dfrac{x}{13 lbs} = \dfrac{\frac{1}{4}mg}{1lb}$

55. $\dfrac{n}{21 lbs} = \dfrac{1cc}{5 lbs}$

56. $\dfrac{23mg}{x} = \dfrac{40mg}{1cc}$

57. $\dfrac{2.4mg}{x} = \dfrac{6mg}{1ml}$

Chapter 9
Measurement Systems

Technicians need to be familiar with a variety of laboratory equipment – graduated cylinders of various sizes, syringes and different types of tips and needles, eyedroppers and other glassware used for preparing, mixing and dispensing medicines and chemicals used in the practice of veterinary medicine. Measuring devices come in a variety of shapes and sizes. It is important to pick an appropriately sized container and measure accurately.

Reading and recording results from measurements are equally important. Great care must be taken when reading graduated cylinders and measuring devices such as spectrometers. The technician should read a device at eye level. Do not raise the item to your level, rather place the item on a flat surface and get down to look at it directly.

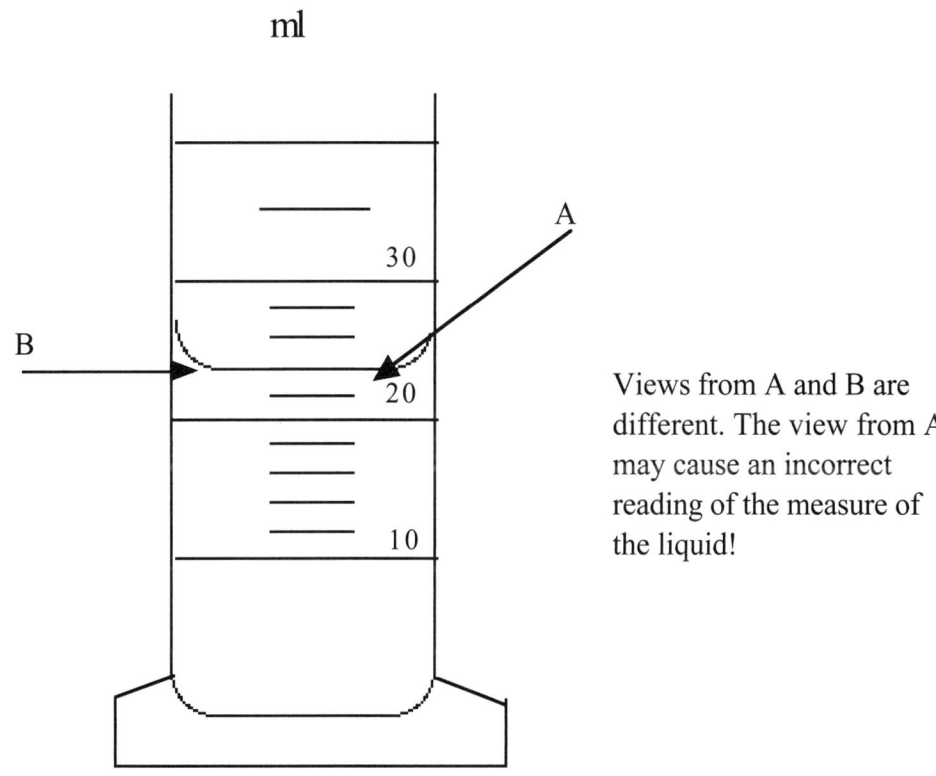

Views from A and B are different. The view from A may cause an incorrect reading of the measure of the liquid!

Common errors that occur when measuring chemicals or medicines include the phenomena of Parallax. *Parallax* is the apparent displacement of an object when viewed from two different points.

130   Measurement Systems

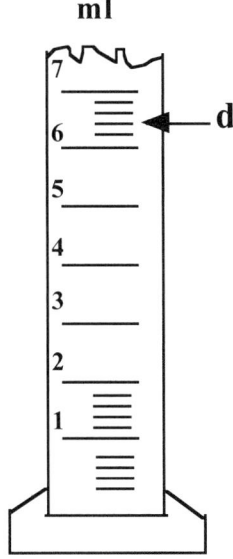

Measurements must also take into account the scale of the container. In this case, the numbers are in milliliters and the marks indicate an increase by "twos" from milliliter to milliliter. Shown (d) is the measure for 6.4 ml.

A liquid wets the container it is in and causes a rise along the contact surface. The portion of the liquid not in contact with the surface does not rise. This capillary action can be seen in a graduated cylinder. The result is a curved upper surface of a liquid column called the meniscus. The *meniscus* is the concave, or curved up at the ends, surface of the liquid measurement. The correct reading is taken along the bottom of the depression.

Another interesting effect is known as capillary action. *Capillary action* is when liquid is pulled up a surface with which it is in contact. If a fine bore tube is inserted into a container of liquid, the level of liquid in the tube will be higher than its level in the surrounding liquid in the container. The finer the bore of the tube, the higher the liquid will be drawn.

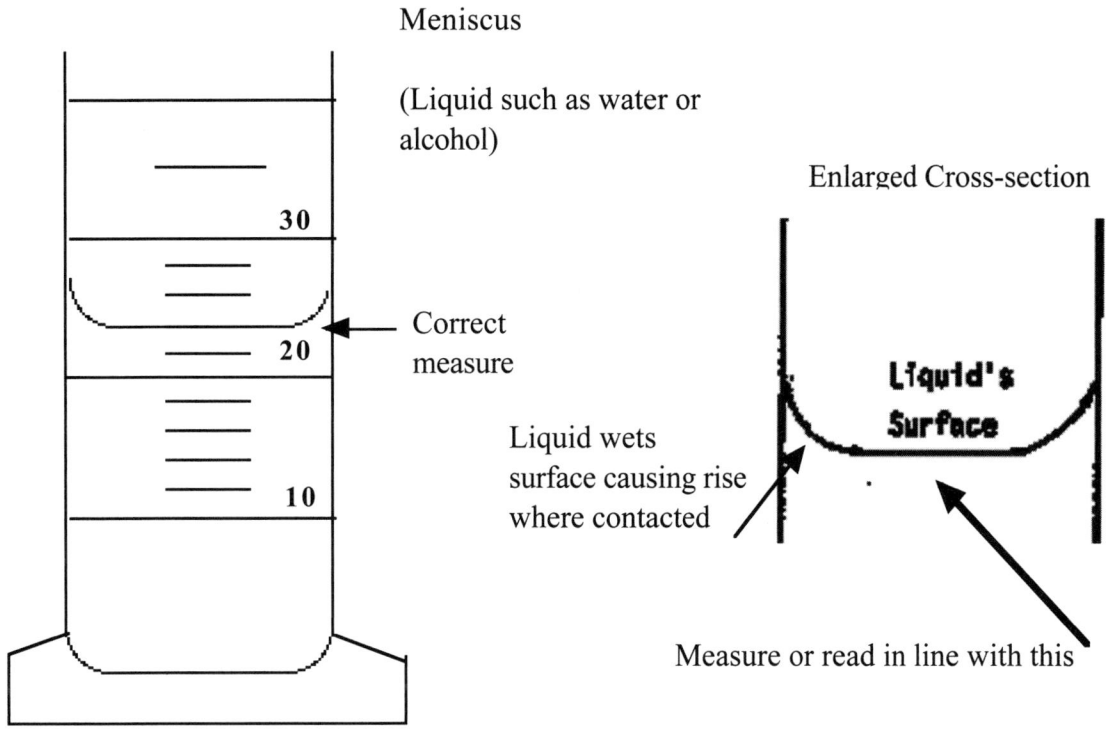

Reading a graduated cylinder with meniscus can result in an error in measurement. Always read straight across the cylinder, lining up the marked measurements along the outside of the cylinder with the bottom of the meniscus.

An error can occur when reading instrument scales. If a scale is viewed off-center, the reading may be incorrect. Most instruments have a reflective strip that allows the reader to hide the reflection of the needle directly behind the needle itself, thus assuring you are correctly reading the instrument.

The technician should be equally aware of common terms likely to be encountered in a clinic or lab such as density and specific gravity.

Density is defined as the amount of mass (or weight) per unit volume. For example,

$$\frac{grams}{milliliter} \qquad \frac{kilogram}{liter} \qquad \frac{lbs}{foot^3}$$

abbreviations can include: g/ml, g/cc, kg/L, lb/ft³

The density of lead is greater than the density of water which indicates that the mass per unit volume of lead is greater than the mass per unit of volume of water.

Specific gravity is a means of comparing densities to that of water. Note that specific gravity is a number with no units.

$$\text{Specific gravity} = \frac{\text{Density of a substance}}{\text{Density of water}}$$

Examples:

(i) $\text{Specific gravity of Lead} = \dfrac{11.3 \text{ g/cc}}{1 \text{ g/cc}} = 11.3$

(ii) $\text{Specific gravity of urine} = \dfrac{1.035 \text{ g/cc}}{1 \text{ g/cc}} = 1.035$

Practice Set IX – 1

1. 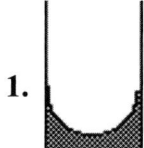 This curved surface of the liquid is called a _____

2. Water can be pulled up a fine bored tube by _____

3. The density of water is _____ g / cc or _____ lb / ft³ .

4. The density of gold is 19.3 g / cc, determine its specific gravity.

5. The density of silver is 10.5 g / cc. Find the specific gravity of silver.

The Metric System

The metric system of measurement is the most widely used system in the world. It is a measurement system based upon powers of ten. The basic units of measurement are the meter for length, the liter for volume, and the gram for mass (weight). Multiples and fractional parts are formed by adding a prefix to the basic unit. The prefixes most commonly used are presented here.

Decimal System	Numerical meaning	Metric Prefix	Abbreviation
Million	1,000,000	Mega-	M
Thousand	1,000	kilo-	k
Hundred	100	hecto-	h
Ten	10	deka-	da
Unit	1	None	None
Tenth	0.1	deci-	d
Hundredth	0.01	centi-	c
Thousandth	0.001	milli-	m
Millionth	0.000001	micro-	μ
Billionth	0.000000001	nano-	n
Trillionth	1×10^{-12}	pico-	p

Practice Set IX – 2

Write the appropriate metric prefix:

1. Hundreds   _____

2. Tenths   _____

3. Units   _____

4. Thousands   _____

5. Thousandths   _____

6. Tens   _____

7. Hundredths   _____

Common abbreviations along with the words for mass, length and volume are given in the chart below. A special note: the abbreviation for deka- has changed several times over the years. The student should be aware that s/he may encounter such variations as decameter (dam), decagram (dag) and decaliter (dal). We will use deka– , unless otherwise noted.

Prefix	Length	Weight	Volume
kilo-	kilometer (km)	kilogram (kg)	kiloliter (kl)
hecto-	hectometer (hm)	hectogram (hg)	hectoliter (hl)
deka-	dekameter (dkm)	dekagram (dkg)	dekaliter (dkl)
basic unit	meter (m)	gram (g)	liter (l)
deci-	decimeter (dm)	decigram (dg)	deciliter (dl)
centi-	centimeter (cm)	centigram (cg)	centiliter (cl)
milli-	millimeter (mm)	milligram (mg)	milliliter (ml)
micro-	micrometer (μm)	microgram (μg)	microliter (μl)

The ability to recreate the following chart will prove to be an invaluable aid in mastering the Metric System and for making conversions within this system.

Measurement Systems

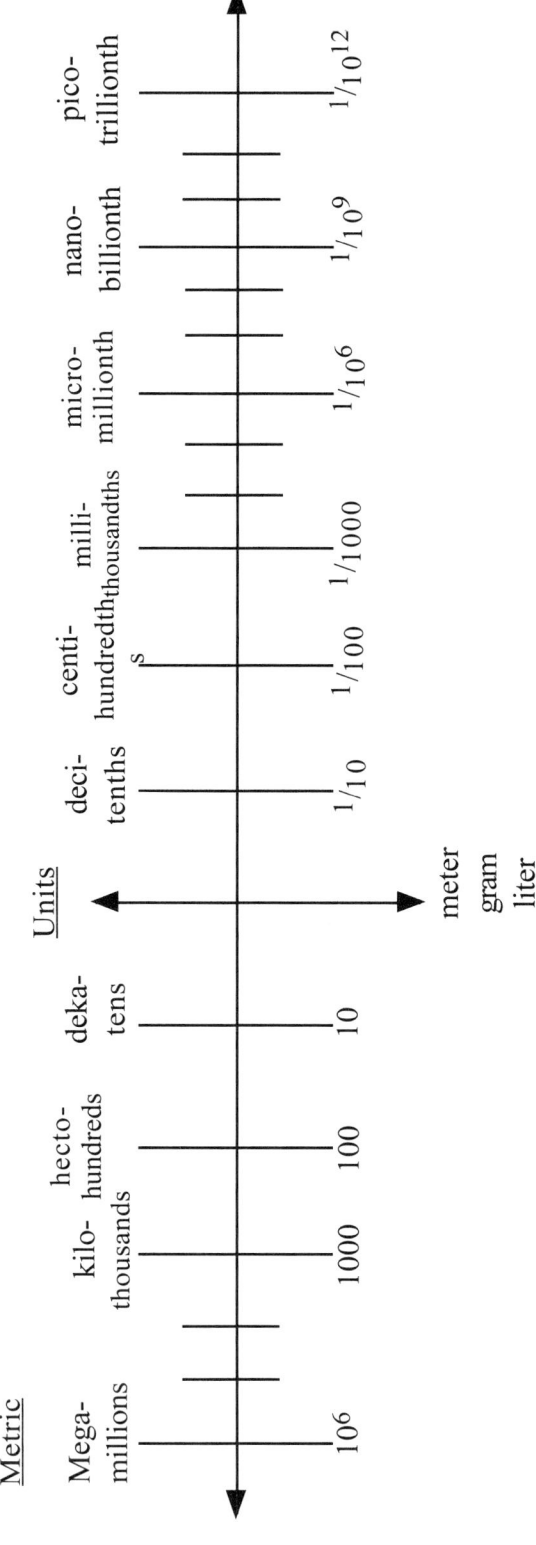

Practice Set IX – 3

Write the abbreviation and the value of the number of units for each of the following.

Metric Units	Abbreviation	Value
kilometer	km	1000 meters
1. decimeter	_____	_____
2. milligram	_____	_____
3. dekagram	_____	_____
4. meter	_____	_____
5. deciliter	_____	_____
6. dekameter	_____	_____
7. gram	_____	_____
8. hectometer	_____	_____
9. decigram	_____	_____
10. centiliter	_____	_____
11. liter	_____	_____
12. dekaliter	_____	_____
13. hectoliter	_____	_____
14. kiloliter	_____	_____
15. milliliter	_____	_____
16. centimeter	_____	_____

Conversion from one metric unit to another

Conversion from one unit to another involves merely moving the decimal point the same number of "steps" in the same direction as it takes to get from one unit to the other.

Examples: (i) 8 km = __?__ cm

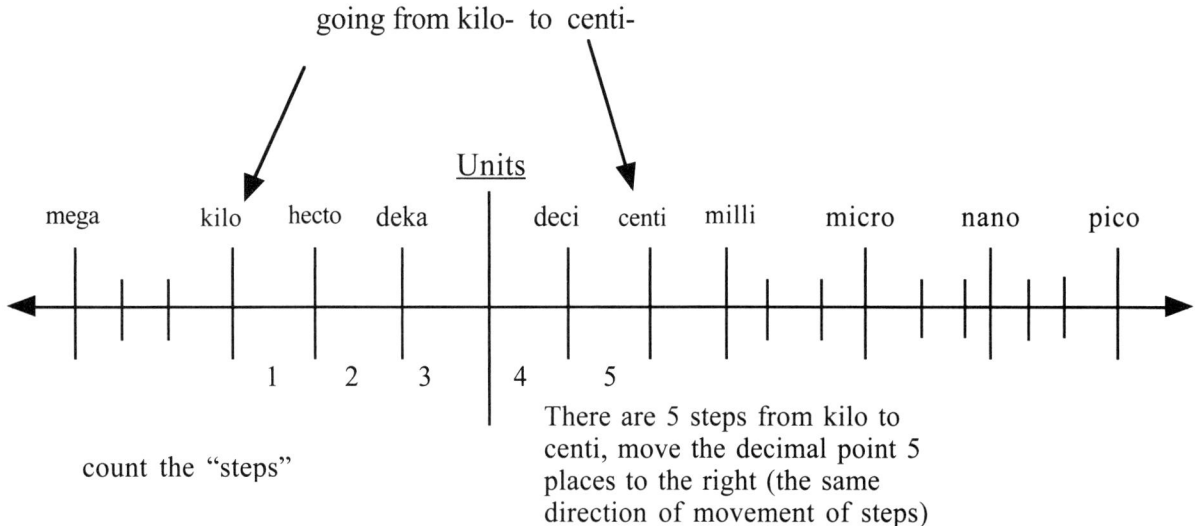

Thus, 8 km = 800000 cm

(ii) 4000.2 mg = ? kg

That's six steps to the left. Move the decimal point the same 6 places to left.

4000.2 mg = ? kg
⬅
move 6 places in this direction

Result? 0.0040002 kg

Note: between milli- and micro-, micro- and nano-, nano- and pico-, mega- and kilo-, there are two unnamed units that must each be considered (counted) as steps.

Practice Set IX – 4

Determine the conversion from one unit to another for each of the following.

1. 0.12 km = _____ dm

2. 12.0 g = _____ mg

3. 0.21 hl = _____ cl

4. 1.5 cm = _____ mm

5. 5.51 dkg = _____ cg

6. 0.6125 hg = _____ mg

7. 3.0 kl = _____ L

8. 401.0 L = _____ cl

9. 515.12 dkl = _____ ml

10. 12.14 km = _____ m

11. 11.2 mg = _____ dg

12. 2.1 dl = _____ kl

13. 12.3 mm = _____ m

14. 51 g = _____ kg

15. 23.5 cm = _____ dkm

16. 65.3 L = _____ hl

17. 3.4 m = _____ km

18. 63.5 dm = _____ dkm

19. 151123.5 ml = _____ kl

Apothecary and English Measurement Systems
Inter– and Intra–System Conversions

Medicines, and other materials, are sometimes measured using an antiquated system called the Apothecaries' system. It is essential for veterinary medical technologists to be as familiar with this system as with the Metric and English systems since each of these systems of measurement are likely to be encountered in the laboratory, office, or clinic.

The following are common units and abbreviations of length, volume, and weight in English and Apothecary systems of measurements.

Length	Volume	Weight
Inches – in	Fluid Ounces – fl. oz.	Grains – gr
Feet – ft	Pints – pts	Ounces – oz
Yards – yds	Quarts – qts	Pounds – lbs
Miles – mi	Gallons – gal	Tons – T

There are also common household measurements with which you should be familiar.

Cups – c   Tablespoons – Tbs or Tbsp or T   Teaspoons – tsp; or t

Equivalents

Length

12 in = 1 ft
36 in = 1 yd
3 ft = 1 yd
5,280 ft = 1 mi

Weight

16 oz = 1 lb
2000 lb = 1 ton

Volume

16 oz = 1 pt
32 fl oz = 1 qt
2 pt = 1 qt
4 qt = 1 gal
8 pt = 1 gal
128 fl oz = 1 gal

1 pt = 2 cups
1 qt = 4 cups
2 Tbs = 1 fl oz
3 tsp = 1 Tbs
6 tsp = 1 fl oz
1 cup = 8 fl oz

Temperature Conversions

$$C = \frac{5}{9}(F - 32)$$
or
$$C = (F - 32) \div 1.8$$

$$F = \frac{9}{5}C + 32$$
or
$$F = 1.8C + 32$$

Approximate Equivalents Between Systems

1 g = 15 gr
65 mg = 1 gr
30 g = 1 oz
454 g = 1 lb
1 kg = 2.2 lb
1 oz = 438 gr

1 cup = 237 ml
1 fl oz = 30 ml
1 tsp = 5 cc
1 pt = 473 ml
1 qt = 946 ml
1 gal = 3.785 L
1 Tbs = 15 ml

1 in = 2.5 cm
1 m = 39.4 in
1 m = 1.09 yd

Measurement Systems

Practice Set IX – 5

Write the abbreviation or the name for each of the following.

1. pint _____
2. T _____
3. cup _____

4. lb _____
5. t _____
6. mile _____

7. oz _____
8. fluid ounce _____
9. ounces _____

10. yard _____
11. gallon _____
12. qt _____

13. inch _____
14. feet _____
15. grains _____

Sometimes it is necessary to convert from one unit to another within a system. Unlike the metric system, this conversion can be difficult and laborious. Since it is not based on unit of ten, the decimal point cannot be moved to obtain the answer. One must use ratio and proportion or conversion factors to convert units.

Example: Convert 2.5 gal into qt

1 gal = 4 qt

ratio / proportion

$$\frac{x\,qt}{2.5\,gal} = \frac{4\,qt}{1\,gal}$$

$$x\,qt = \frac{4\,qt \times 2.5\,gal}{1\,gal}$$

$$x = 10\,qt$$

conversion

conversion factor: $\frac{4\,qt}{1\,gal}$

$$x = 2.5\,gal\left(\frac{4\,qt}{1\,gal}\right)$$

$$x = 10\,qt$$

Examples:

(i) Convert 7 pts to cups. 2 cups = 1 pt

$$\frac{7 \text{ pints}}{} \bigg| \frac{2 \text{ cups}}{1 \text{ pint}} = 14 \text{ cups} \qquad 7 \text{ pints is equal to 14 cups}$$

(ii) Convert 2.5 gals to fluid ounces. 128 fl oz = 1 gal

$$\frac{2.5 \text{ gal}}{} \bigg| \frac{128 \text{ fl oz}}{1 \text{ gal}} = 320 \text{ fl oz}$$

(iii) Convert 2.5 days into minutes. 1 day = 24 hrs, 1 hr = 60 min

$$\frac{2.5 \text{ days}}{} \bigg| \frac{24 \text{ hr}}{1 \text{ day}} \bigg| \frac{60 \text{ min}}{1 \text{ hr}} = 3600 \text{ min}$$

Practice Set IX – 6

Convert the following into the desired units. Use any method.

1. 2.5 gal = _____ qts

2. 256 fl oz = _____ gal

3. 6 T = _____ t

4. 27 fl oz = _____ T

5. 5 pts = _____ c

6. 2.5 lbs. = _____ oz

7. $2\frac{1}{4}$ ft = _____ in

8. $4\frac{1}{3}$ yd = _____ ft

9. 18 fl oz = _____ tsp

10. 14 ft = _____ in

11. 3 oz = _____ gr.

12. 1.5 qt = _____ fl oz

13. 2 mi = _____ ft

14. 1.7 tons = _____ lbs.

15. 3 tablespoons = _____ tsp

16. 25 oz = _____ lbs.

Practice Set IX – 7

Convert. Use any method.

1. 16 fl oz _____ pts

2. 32 fl oz _____ pts _____ qts

3. 128 fl oz _____ pts _____ qts _____ gals

4. 3 gals _____ qts _____ pts _____ fl oz

5. 16 oz _____ lbs.

6. 3 lbs. _____ oz

7. 6 ft _____ in

_____ **Measurement Systems** 145

8. 36 ft _____ yds

9. 7 in _____ ft

10. 72 oz _____ lbs.

11. 3 Tbsp _____ fl oz

12. 1 Tbsp _____ tsp

13. 1 tsp _____ T

14. 30 fl oz _____ tsp

15. 30 fl oz _____ tablespoons

16. 8 oz _____ lbs.

17. 24 lbs. _____ oz

18. 10 Tbsp _____ tsp

It is often necessary to convert from the metric to the English or apothecaries' systems (or back). For example, if an animal is weighed in pounds and the dosage is in kilograms.

Measurement Systems

Generally, the equivalents used for everyday simple tasks are not as accurate as shown. Frequently, for example, liters and quarts are considered equivalent. For some non-critical applications this may be acceptable. However, the use of such rough apporximations is not acceptable in scientific or research work.

Examples:

(i) Actual   Common rough approximation
     1 qt. = 946 ml   1 qt = 1000 ml = 1 L

(ii) It may be common to use the following measures for cups/milliliters

1 cup = 237 ml   and   1 pt = 500 ml   but   1 pt = 2 cups

Of course, there is no substitute for good judgment. One should not convert gallons to milliliters and then the milliliters to fluid ounces (*inter*system.)

It is easier, more efficient, and more accurate to convert directly from gallons to fluid ounces (*intra–system*).

$$1 \text{ gal} = 128 \text{ fl oz}$$

Still, there are occasions when you must convert from one value to another, from one system to another, or even make several conversions at a time. However, this should be done only as a last resort or when no better alternative is available. A liter and a quart, for instance, are generally considered approximately equivalent for quick conversions.

Q.   1 L = ??? tsp

A.   *1 L = 1000 ml = 200 tsp*

The conversion from one system to another can be done in three ways: ratios and proportions; dimensional analysis; or, if available, simple conversion factors.

Example: Convert 2.5 liters to gallons

Ratio and Proportion

$$\frac{x}{2.5\ L} = \frac{1\ gal}{3.785\ L}$$

$$x = \frac{2.5\ L \cdot 1\ gal}{3.785\ L}$$

$x = 0.66$ gal

Conversion Factor

$$x = 2.5\ L \left(\frac{1\ gal}{3.785\ L}\right)$$

$x = 0.66$ gal

Dimensional analysis

$$\frac{2.5\ \cancel{liters} \mid 1\ gallon}{\mid 3.785\ \cancel{L}} = 0.66\ gallons$$

Measurement Systems

The use of dimensional analysis shows it is a useful technique for keeping track of the proper units when doing a problem. Dimensional analysis is commonly used in chemistry.

Examples: (i) Change 74 pounds to kilograms

$$\frac{74 \text{ lb} \mid 1 \text{ kg}}{\mid 2.2 \text{ lb}} = \frac{74 \text{ kg}}{2.2} = \frac{74}{2.2} kg \approx 33.6 \ kg$$

(ii) 25 g/100 ml rewritten in terms of milligrams is

$$\frac{25 \text{ g} \mid \overset{10}{\cancel{1000}} \text{ mg}}{\cancel{100} \text{ ml} \mid 1 \text{ g}} = 250 \ mg/ml$$

(iii) Convert 75 grains into ounces.

$$\frac{75 \text{ gr} \mid 1 \text{ oz}}{\mid 438 \text{ gr}} = 0.17 \text{ oz}$$

Practice Set IX – 8

Convert. Use proportions or dimensional analysis.

1. 35 ml = _____ tsp

2. 4.5 L = _____ gal

3. 5 in = _____ cm

4. $3\frac{1}{2}$ fl oz = _____ cc

5. 2700 ml = _____ qt

6. 3 Tbs. = _____ cc

7. 45 g = _____ oz

8. 2.4 gr. = _____ mg

9. 3 g = _____ gr.

10. 27 kg = _____ lbs.

11. 2 lb = _____ g

12. 3 m = _____ in

Temperature Conversion

The two most common temperature scales are *Celsius* and *Fahrenheit*.

To convert from Fahrenheit to Celsius: $C = \frac{5}{9}(F - 32)$ or $C = (F - 32)/1.8$

To convert from Celsius to Fahrenheit: $F = \frac{9}{5}C + 32$ or $F = 1.8C + 32$

Measurement Systems

The boiling point of water is 212° F or 100° C. Each of these represents the same temperature needed to boil water. Each merely represents a different scale of measurement. The freezing point of water is 32° F or 0° C. Both describe the same condition with regards to heat (or lack of heat = cold.)

To convert from one temperature scale to another, use the given formula, substitute the known value and simplify.

Examples:

F → C

70° F = ? C

$$C = \frac{5}{9}(70° - 32°)$$

$$C = 21.1°$$

C → F

18° C = ? F

$$F = \frac{9}{5}(18°) + 32°$$

$$F = 64.4°$$

Practice Set IX – 9

Convert (round to nearest tenth degree where necessary):

1. 40° C = _____ °F

2. 60° F = _____ °C

3. 37° C = _____ °F

4. 65° F = _____ °C

5. 32° F = _____ °C

6. 70° F = _____ °C

_____ Measurement Systems

7. 45° C = _____ °F   8. 73° F = _____ °C

9. 100° F = _____ °C   10. 78° C = _____ °F

11. 0° F = _____ °C   12. 80° C = _____ °F

13. −40° C = _____ °F   14. 100° C = _____ °F

15. −10° F = _____ °C   16. 80° F = _____ °C

17. 25° C = _____ °F   18. 50° C = _____ °F

19. 10° F = _____ °C   20. 18° C = _____ °F

Practice Set IX – 10

Convert as indicated (round to hundredths if necessary):

1. 3 g = _____ gr.   2. 5 oz = _____ g

3. 130 mg = _____ gr.   4. 4.5 oz = _____ g

Measurement Systems

5. 3 oz = _____ g

6. 35 ml = _____ tsp

7. $2\frac{1}{2}$ lbs. = _____ g

8. 5 lb = _____ kg

9. 2.5 cups = _____ cc

10. 8 fl oz = _____ ml

11. 4 tsp = _____ ml

12. 3 pts = _____ ml

13. 7.5 pts = _____ L

14. 45 ml = _____ Tbs.

15. 12 in = _____ cm

16. 350 g = _____ lbs.

17. 45 g = _____ oz

18. 55 ml = _____ fl oz

19. 100 ml = _____ fl oz

20. 3 tsp = _____ ml

21. 3 Tbs. = _____ ml   **22.** 5 pts = _____ L

23. 85 ml = _____ tsp   **24.** 85 ml = _____ Tbs.

25. 15 ml = _____ tsp   **26.** 45 gr. = _____ oz

27. 100 g = _____ oz   **28.** 300 mg = _____ gr.

29. 13 g = _____ gr.   **30.** 220 gr. = _____ g

Practice Set IX – 11
Convert. Round to two places, if necessary.

1. 32 oz = _____ lbs.   **2.** 18 pts = _____ qts

3. 16 pts = _____ gal   **4.** 6 tsp = _____ Tbs.

5. 8 tsp = _____ ml   **6.** 1 gal = _____ ml

Measurement Systems

7. 5 tsp = _____ Tbs.

8. 3 cups = _____ fl oz

9. 3 pts = _____ cups

10. 12 cups = _____ pts

11. 100 ml = _____ Tbs.

12. 1 cup = _____ fl oz

13. 5 ml = _____ tsp

14. 3 oz = _____ g

15. 10 ml = _____ Tbs.

16. 3 gr. = _____ mg

17. 500 ml = _____ pts

18. 5 g = _____ gr.

19. 1000 ml = _____ pts

20. $1\frac{1}{2}$ g = _____ gr.

21. 12 L = _____ qts

22. 7 ml = _____ tsp

23. 200 ml = _____ qts

24. $2\frac{1}{2}$ fl oz = _____ Tbs.

25. 6 pts = _____qts

26. 150 mg = _____gr

27. 13 qts = _____gal

28. 48 g = _____ oz

29. 12 ml = _____tsp

30. 85 gr. = _____g

31. 12 ml = _____Tbs.

32. 30 ml = _____Tbs.

33. 750 ml = _____ pts

34. 145 g = _____oz

35. 5 oz = _____g

36. 6 qts = _____fl oz

37. 2 fl oz = _____ml

38. 5 tsp = _____ml

39. 7 Tbs. = _____ ml

40. 1.5 tsp = _____ml

Practice Set IX – 12

Convert. Round to hundredths, if necessary.

1. 5 cg = _____ g

2. 1 g = _____ mg

3. 2 cups = _____ pints = _____ qts = _____ cc

4. 11 pints = _____ qts

5. 500 cc = _____ liters

6. 2.5 L = _____ ml = _____ cc

7. 0.25 L = _____ ml

8. 0.1 g = _____ mg

9. 1 fl oz = _____ ml

Measurement Systems 157

10. 1 qt = _____ fl oz

11. 1 g = _____ grains

12. 4 cups = _____ cc = _____ pts = _____ qts

13. 5 cc = _____ tsp

14. 1 g = _____ mg

15. 6 fl oz = _____ cc

16. 2 kg = _____ lbs.

17. 150 mg = _____ g

18. 1 gr. = _____ mg

19. 1 gal = _____ qts = _____ pts = _____ cc

20. 8 g = _____ mg

Measurement Systems

21. 0.5 g = _____ mg

22. 600 cc = _____ L

23. 250 mg = _____ g

24. 1000 mg = _____ g

25. 15 g = _____ cg

26. 11 kg = _____ lbs.

27. 1000 cc = _____ L

28. 32 fl oz = _____ qt

29. 2 g = _____ gr.

30. 4000 cc = _____ gal

31. 4 pts = _____ qts

Unit III

Chapter 10
Dosage and Concentration Applications
Using Ratios and Proportions

Understanding and solving word problems involves some of the most critical skills a technician can learn. We communicate both orally and with the written word as we work together in an office or clinic. The doctor who asks for 3 cc of atropine for an injection, for instance, trusts the technician to supply exactly that. The calculation of dosages is a critical area — it must be done quickly and accurately. The dosage is the required amount to administer for a particular patient for a specific result. The concentration is the potentcy of the medicine – the amount of medicine, or active ingredient.

When solving word problems, there are several principles that are useful:
- Decide what is being asked. What is needed for the result?
- Catalog the information given - write it down!
- Determine the ratio and proportions needed, including the units.

Example: A dose of sodium pentobarbital is needed for a 125 pound dog. The dosage given on the label is 1 cc per 5 pounds of body weight.

1. What is needed? – the amount to administer to the dog is "x" cc.

2. Known information: dosage of $\dfrac{1cc}{5lbs}$ and weight of dog – 125 pounds.

3. Determine the appropriate proportion: $\dfrac{Xcc}{125lbs} = \dfrac{1cc}{5lbs}$

4. Solve: $\dfrac{Xcc}{125lbs} = \dfrac{1cc}{5lbs}$ the lbs units cancel; 5 divides evenly into 125

$$Xcc = \dfrac{\cancel{125}^{25}lbs \times 1cc}{\cancel{5}_{1}lbs}$$

$$X = 25cc$$

The correct dosage for the 125 pound dog is 25 cc.

162   Dosage and Concentration Applications

Using dimensional analysis:

$$\frac{1 \text{ cc}}{\cancel{5} \cancel{\text{lbs}}_1} \bigg| \frac{\cancel{125 \text{ pounds}}^{25}}{} = 25 \text{ cc}$$

Pound units cancel and 5 divides into 125 evenly ("cancels")

(ii) An 11 pound cat is prescribed a dosage of medicine with a concentration of 100 mg per 5 pounds. How many milligrams should be administered?

$$\frac{\cancel{100}^{20} \text{ mg}}{\cancel{5} \cancel{\text{lbs}}_1} \bigg| \frac{11 \cancel{\text{lbs}}}{} = 220 \text{ mg}$$

Practice Set X – 1

Solve the following problems.

1. How much Surital is needed for a dog weighing 25 pounds if the dosage is 1 cc per 5 pounds of body weight?

2. How much Surital would be necessary if the dog weighed 67 pounds?

3. A tranquilizer, Nortron, can be used at the rate of 4 mg per 1 pound of body weight. How much is needed for a 40 pound dog?

4. How much ketomine is necessary for a 10 pound cat if the dosage is 15 mg per 1 lb.

5. If a 10 lb dog requires 2.5 cc of medication, how many cc will a 25 lb dog require?

Dosage and Concentration Applications 163

Some medicines in the veterinary clinic are prescribed in milligrams per pound of body weight, yet they're packaged in milligrams per cc. To compute the proper dosage requires multiple steps:

- calculate the number of mg to be given for a particular weight of animal
- calculate the number of cc which contains the number of mg computed

Example: Ketomine is given at the dosage of 15 mg per 1 lb body weight. It is packaged in the bottle at a concentration of 100 mg per 1 cc. How many cc should be given to a 27 lb cat?

(i) Determine the amount of ketomine in mg based upon the 27 lb cat.

$$\frac{x}{27 lbs} = \frac{15 mg}{1 lbs} \quad \text{cross-multiply and simplify}$$

$$x = \frac{27 lbs \times 15 mg}{1 lbs}$$

$$x = 405 mg$$

(ii) This gives the amount of medicine necessary. Determine the cc equivalent.

$$\frac{405 mg}{x} = \frac{100 mg}{1 cc} \quad \text{solve the proportion by cross-multiplying and simplifying}$$

$$x = \frac{405 mg \times 1 cc}{100 mg}$$

$$x = 4.05 \ cc$$

Same problem using dimensional analysis.

$$\frac{15 \ mg}{1 \ lb} \left| \frac{27 \ lb}{} \right| \frac{1 \ cc}{100 \ mg} = \frac{405}{100} cc = 4.05 \ cc$$

Practice Set X – 2

1. How many cc of ketomine should be administered to a 17 pound cat when the doctor has prescribed a dosage of 15 mg per pound of body weight? The ketomine is packaged in a concentration of 100 mg per 1 cc.

2. Phenobarbital is given to a dog at the rate of 3 mg per pound of body weight. The dog weighs 42 pounds. The concentration is 50 mg per cc. How many cc should be administered?

3. Prednisaolone is prescribed in a dosage of 0.5 mg / lb. for a 15 pound dog. How many cc are necessary if the concentration is 5 mg per cc?

4. Sulfamethazine is to be given to a 30 pound dog at the rate of 25 mg / lb. How many cc are necessary if the concentration is 200 mg per cc?

5. Morphine has been prescribed at the rate of 1 mg / 15 lb for a 125 pound dog. The concentration is 10 mg per cc. How many cc should be administered?

Practice Set X – 3

Solve the following using ratio and proportion techniques. (B.W. = body weight)

1. Surital can be used as an anesthetic in a dosage of 1 cc per 5 lbs B.W. How much should be used in each of the following cases:

   a. For a 15 lb cat?   b. For a 65 lb Boxer?

2. Surital can also be used as an anesthetic in a dosage of 1 cc per 3 lbs B.W. How much should be used for each of the animals in (1) ?

3. To reduce salivation when using Surital, atropine can be used in a dosage of 1 cc per 25 lb B.W. How much should be used for each of the animals in (1) ?

4. Ketomine can be used an an intramuscular anesthetic for cats. The dosage is 15 mg per pound of B.W.
   a. How much should be administered to a 12 pound cat?

   b. The ketomine comes dissolved in a liquid at 100 mg per cc. How many cc must be given for the prescribed dosage in part (a)?

5. Amphesol (5%) is given as a stimulant at a dosage of 0.4 ml per 10 lbs B.W. How much is needed to stimulate a 35 pound dog?

6. A tranquilizer, Nortran, is given to animals at the dosage of $1/4$ mg per lb B.W.

   a. How many mg will be needed for a female dog of 45 pounds in order to tranquilize her?

   b. The Nortran is packaged in tablets of 10 mg each. Determine the nearest whole number of tablets needed for (**a**)

7. A different tranquilizer, Jenoton, is administered at the rate of 1.5 mg per lb of B.W.

   a. How much is required for a 125 lb dog?

   b. If the medication is packaged as a 25 mg per cc concentration, how many cc are needed?

8. A boxer weighing 53 pounds has hook worms. DNP (45 mg/ml) is prescribed at the rate of 0.1 cc per lb of B.W. How much should be administered?

Practice Set X – 4

1. A dog weighing 35 pounds needs atropine sulfate ($1/120$ grain per cc) at the rate of 1 cc per 25 lbs B.W. How many cc are needed?

2. Surital (5%) can be used as an anesthetic at a dosage of 1 cc per 5 lbs B.W. How many cc are needed for each of the following:

    a. 6 lb cat   **b.** 9 lb cat   **c.** 73 lb dog

    d. 35 lb dog   **e.** 18 lb dog

3. Surital (5%) used as an anesthetic is packaged in solution 1 cc per 3 lbs B.W. How many cc are needed for each of the animals in (**2.**)?

Dosage and Concentration Applications

4. Ketomine is an intramuscular anesthetic for cats at a dosage of 15 mg per lb B.W. The ketomine is dissolved in a liquid at 100 mg per cc. How many cc are needed for each of the following cats:

a. 6 lb   **b.** 8.5 lb   **c.** 18 lb   **d.** 13 lb

5. A tranquilizer, Nortran, is used at the rate of $1/4$ mg per lb of B.W. Determine the amount necessary for each of the following dogs:

a. 36 lb   **b.** 125 lb   **c.** 25 lb   **d.** 73 lb

6. The tranquilizer, Jenoton, is used at a rate of 1.5 mg per lb B.W. How much would be needed for each of the animals in (**5.**)?

7. DNP used for hookworms is prescribed at 0.1 cc per lb B.W. What is the dosage for each of the animals in (**5**)?

Practice Set X – 5

   1. Pentobarbital is administered to a dog which weighs 35 pounds. The dosage rate is 1 cc per 5 lb B.W.   **a.** What is the total amount to be administered?

   b. Only 60% is to be given immediately. How many cc will this be?

   c. Shown is a 12 cc syringe. Assume that the syringe is filled with the amount calculated in (i). Indicate by an arrow (↓) on the syringe where this would be. Indicate using a double arrow (↓↓) the point where the medication would be discharged to administer the initial 60%.

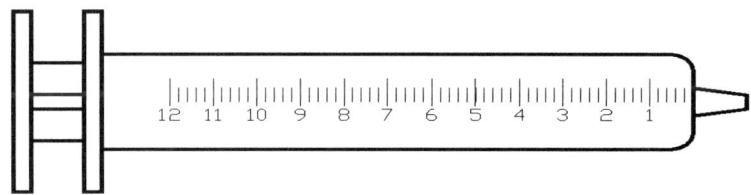

   2. Pentobarbital is to be administered to a 47 pound dog. The dosage is 1 cc per 5 lb.
   a. What is the total amount needed?

   b. If 60% is administered initially, How many cc are needed?

   c. Shown is a 12 cc syringe. Assume that the syringe is filled with the amount calculated in (i). Indicate by an arrow (↓) on the syringe where this would be. Indicate using a double arrow (↓↓) the point where the medication would be discharged to administer the initial 60%.

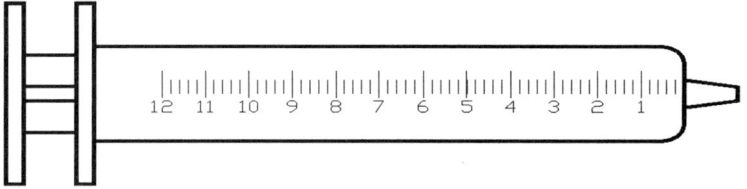

170   Dosage and Concentration Applications

3. Pentobarbital is prescribed for a dog which weighs 15 lbs. The dosage is 1 cc per 5 lb.

    a. What is the total amount of the prescribed dose?

    b. 60% is to be administered initially. How many cc will that take?

    c. Shown is a 12 cc syringe. Assume that the syringe is filled with the amount calculated in (i). Indicate by an arrow (↓) on the syringe where this would be. Indicate using a double arrow (↓↓) the point where the medication would be discharged to administer the initial 60%.

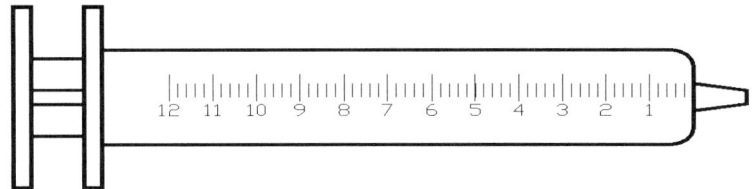

Solutions that are prepared from concentrations can be made by determining the value of the percent of concentration and changing this to grams. Dissolve the appropriate gram amount in water to make 100 ml of the correct concentration of the needed solution.

Review of terms

       % means parts per 100

       grams% means grams per 100 ml

   Thus, the term % can represent either grams per 100 ml or ml per 100 ml

Dosage and Concentration Applications 171

Solutions used in practices can be formulated as needed. Dissolving a salt in distilled water, for instance, will make a saline solution. The concentration of the solution determines the amount of chemical necessary.

Examples: (i) Prepare 600 ml of an 8% saline solution. $8\% \rightarrow \dfrac{8\ g}{100\ ml}$

Form a proportion and solve.
$$\dfrac{8\ g}{100\ ml} = \dfrac{x\ g}{600\ ml}$$
$$x = 48\ g$$

(ii) Make 1000 ml of a 12% solution.

$$12\% = \dfrac{12\ g}{100\ ml}$$
$$\dfrac{12\ g}{100\ ml} = \dfrac{x}{1000\ ml}$$
$$x = 120\ g$$

Solutions typically have a concentration of chemical to water or alcohol. A 10% solution has 10 parts per 100. Practically that means there are 10 grams of say, salt, dissolved in 100 ml of water.

Example: To make 500 ml of a 10% saline solution dissolve 10 grams of salt per 100 ml. Mathematically...

$$\dfrac{10\ g}{100\ ml} = \dfrac{x}{500\ ml}$$

Solve this proportion for the missing value. To make 500 ml of saline solution of the same 10% concentration, use 50 g of salt.

172   Dosage and Concentration Applications

Example: A 0.9% sodium chloride solution is required. Dissolve 0.9 grams of sodium chloride in 100 ml water to make 100 ml of 0.9% solution.

The problem can be more complex if the desired volume is not 100 ml. For example, how much sodium chloride would be needed to prepare only 60 ml of 0.9% solution?

Solve this problem using the same ratio and proportion methods you have been using.

It is known that: $\frac{0.9g}{100ml}$ but what is needed is $\frac{?g}{60ml}$ in order to achieve the correct concentration.

$$\frac{x}{60ml} = \frac{0.9g}{100ml}$$ cross-multiply and simplify. The ml units cancel

$$x = \frac{0.9g \times 60ml}{100ml}$$

$$x = 0.54g$$

Thus, 0.54 grams of sodium chloride is needed to make 60 ml of 0.9% solution.

Example: A solution is composed of 95 ml of water and 5 ml of formalin. Determine the amount of formalin necessary to make 1000 ml of solution of the same concentration.

Total volume of known solution: 95 ml + 5 ml = 100 ml

For every 100 ml of solution, 5 ml of formalin is needed. Writing as a proportion:

$$\frac{5ml}{100ml} = \frac{x}{1000ml}$$

$$x = \frac{5ml \times 1000ml}{100ml}$$

$$x = 50ml$$

So, 50 ml of formalin is needed to make 1000 ml of the formalin solution.

Dosage and Concentration Applications   173

Practice Set X – 6

1. How many grams of sodium chloride will be needed to prepare 4000 ml of saline solution at 9% concentration?

2. Prepare 4000 ml solution of 5% dextrose.

3. Prepare 1000 ml of 2.5% dextrose.

4. Prepare 500 ml solution of 10% dextrose is needed.

5. Prepare a 3000 ml solution of 5% formalin. (Formalin is measured in ml)

6. Prepare 4000 ml of a solution of 10% formalin solution.

7. Calculate the amount of each chemical needed to make 600 ml of solution if one gram of Iodine and two grams potassium Iodine is used to make 100 ml of solution.

8. If a solution calls for 2 ml Acetic Acid and 98 ml of H_2O, and if 1600 ml of the solution is needed; How much acetic acid should be used?

9. If 1000 ml of a certain solution contains 1.5 g NaCl, how many grams of NaCl are needed to make 1500 ml of the solution?

10. It takes 1 g of mercuric bichloride to make 1200 ml of solution. How many grams of mercuric bichloride would it take to make 750 ml of solution?

11. In making a 2% solution, 16 g of boric acid crystals are dissolved in 800 ml of water. How many grams of boric acid crystals are needed to make 50 ml of solution?

12. To prepare a certain solution, 1 gram of potassium permanganate crystals is added to 5000 ml of water. How many grams of potassium permanganate crystals should be added to 2000 ml of water to make the same concentration of the solution?

13. 100 ml of a solution containing 0.5 g Methylene Blue and 1 ml of Formalin (with a total volume of 100 ml). How much Methylene Blue would be needed to make 1200 ml of solution of the same concentration?

14. A solution is to be made using 1 g of Giemsa in 50 ml of solution. How much of the Giemsa will be needed to make 3000 ml of that solution?

Practice Set X – 7

For each of the following solutions, determine the number of grams (or ml if liquid) are necessary to:

1. Make a 2500 ml solution of saline 0.9%

2. Prepare a 525 ml solution of 2% formalin.

3. Prepare a 650 ml solution of 5% formalin.

4. Prepare 950 ml of 5% dextrose solution.

5. Make 3250 ml of 10% formalin solution.

6. Make 75 ml of NaCl at 0.9%

7. Prepare 25 ml of 1% alcoholic (in alcohol) solution of phenolphthalein.

8. Make 95 ml of 1% copper sulfate.

9. Make 200 ml of 10% Potassium solution.

Dosage and Concentration Applications

10. Prepare 75 ml of a 1% silver nitrate solution.

11. Prepare 35 ml of 1% silver chloride solution.

Calculate the percentage of concentration of a solution by dividing the active ingredient by the volume of diluent.

Examples: (i) 320 ml of ethyl alcohol in 500 ml of solution yields a solution of 64%.

$$\frac{320\ ml}{500\ ml} = 0.64 \rightarrow 64\%$$

(ii) 9 grams of saline salt in 50 ml of solution yields $\frac{9\ g}{50\ ml} = 0.18 = 18\%$

Ignore units when computing the percentage concentration.

Calculate the percentage of solution for each of the following.

12. 190 ml of ethyl alcohol in 200 ml of solution.

13. 3.6 g of sodium chloride in 400 ml of water.

14. 4.5 g of copper sulfate in 225 ml of solution.

15. 15 g of glucose in 300 ml of solution.

16. 4.5 g of sodium chloride in 500 ml of solution.

17. 27 g of sodium chloride in 900 ml of solution.

18. 210 ml of isopropyl alcohol in 300 ml of solution.

Practice Set X – 8

1. Surital can be used as a pre-anesthetic at a dosage of 1 cc per 5 lbs B.W. How much should you use for a 19 lb dog?

2. Surital can also be used as an anesthetic at a dosage of 1 cc per 3 lb B.W. How much should you use for a 25 lb cat?

3. To reduce salivation when using Surital, atropine can be used at a dosage of 1 cc per 20 lb B.W. How much should be used for a 9 lb cat?

4. Ketomine can be used as an intramuscular anesthetic for cats. The dosage is 15 mg per lb of B.W. The ketomine is available in bottled form with a concentration of 100 mg per cc. How many cc are needed for a 14 lb cat?

5. Amphesol (amphetamine sulfate) is given as a stimulant at a dosage of 0.4 ml per 10 lb B.W. How much is needed to stimulate a 30 pound dog?

6. Nortran is given to animals at the dosage of $1/4$ mg per 1 lb B.W. **a.** How much is needed for a 39 lb dog? **b.** Notran comes in tablet form of 10 mg each. What is the nearest whole number of tablets necessary?

7. Jenoton is given at the rate of 1.5 mg per lb B.W. to a 25 lb dog. It is packaged in a 25 mg per 1 cc concentration. How many cc are necessary for the dog?

8. DNP used for hookworms is given at 0.1 cc per lb B.W. How much should be prescribed for a 75 lb dog?

9. Prednisolone is prescribed for a 20 lb dog. The dosage is 0.5 mg per lb and the concentration is 5 mg per cc. How many cc are needed?

10. Morphine has been prescribed at the rate of 2 mg per lb for a 93 lb dog. The concentration is 15 mg per cc. How many cc should you prepare?

11. Make a 2000 ml solution of a normal saline 0.9% solution. How much salt (in grams) will you need to use?

12. To prepare a 590 ml solution of 5% dextrose, how many grams of dextrose would you need?

13. Prepare 85 ml of 0.9% saline. How much NaCl is needed?

14. Make 50 ml of 1% alcoholic solution of phenolphthalein.

15. Prepare 95 ml of 1% copper sulfate solution. How many grams of copper sulfate do you need?

16. Ketomine is used for a 13 lb cat at 15 mg per lb. How many cc are needed if the concentration is 100 mg per cc?

17. Surital is to be given to a 52 lb dog. The dosage is 1 cc per 5 lb. How many cc should you prepare?

18. Phenobarbital is to be administered to a 24 lb dog at the rate of 2 cc / 5 lbs. How much do you need?

19. Morphine is prescribed at 2 mg per lb; the concentration is 15 mg / cc. How many cc do you prepare for a 100 lb dog?

20. Using the label provided, determine the number of milliliters for an 70 lb dog if the recommended dose is 100 mg for 10 pounds B.W.

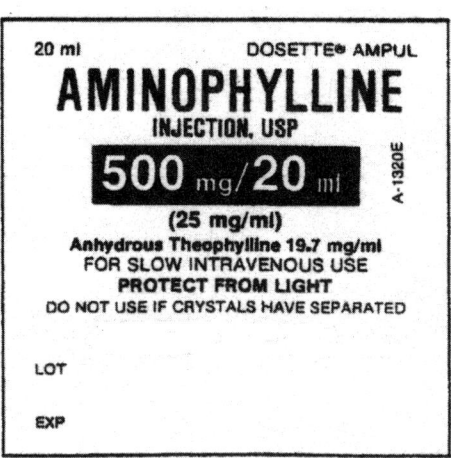

21. Using the label provided, determine the number of cc's needed for a 47 lb dog, if the dosage is 5 mg for 10 lbs B.W.

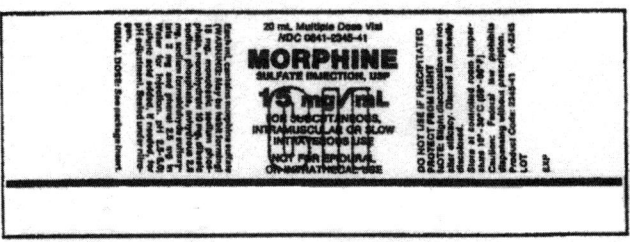

182   Dosage and Concentration Applications

Applications
Dosage and Inter-System Conversion

Whether in the lab or in the clinic, the technician preparing or administering medications must be able to locate the necessary information, determine the concentration, and calculate the proper dosage. For each of the following problems, use the given information to answer the questions.

Example:

A horse with symptoms of pneumonia is to be treated with a sulfa drug. Determine the proper dose(s) for the 900 pound horse.

Drug	Use	Dosage	Species	Patient
(i) sulfadimethoxine 400 mg/ml	for pneumonia	55 mg/kg 1 ml/ 16 lb	horse	900 lb horse

900 lbs. = 409.1 kg

$$\frac{55\ mg}{1\ kg} = \frac{x}{409.1\ kg} \qquad \frac{400\ mg}{1\ ml} = \frac{22500.5\ mg}{x}$$

$$x = 22,500.5\ mg \qquad x = 56.25\ ml$$

The horse should receive a dose of 56.25 ml of the drug at the concentration given.

Practice Set X – 10
   Solve the problem.

Drug	**Use**	**Dosage**	**Species**	**Patient**
1. V-Estravarin Anestrous		0.1 ml/5 lb	dog	35 lb dog
2. Mannitol 20%	CNS injury	1.5 - 2.0 g / kg 8 ml/kg of 20% sol	dogs & cats	4 kg cat
3. Electrosulf-3 (1 lb pkg.)	pneumonia	(in drinking water) 8 oz/25 gal water Use 1 gal medicated water for each 100 lb B.W.. per day for 4 days	calves	150 lb calf

184   Dosage and Concentration Applications

4. Erythro-200 (injection: 200 mg/ml)	pneumonia	2 mg/lb daily	swine	500 lb hog
5. Dextran 6%	plasma expander for shock	up to 200 ml/kg over a period of 24 hours	dogs & cats	55 kg dog
6. Liquamycin (50 mg/ml)	infections	2 mg/ lb	cattle/horses	1100 lb horse
7. Hava Span Boluses	pneumonia	1 bolus/ 100 lb for 6 days (dose lasts 48 hours)	cattle	1200 lb cow

_____ **Dosage and Concentration Applications**   185

Practice Set X – 10
Solve the following problems.

1. Use acepromazine for a preanesthetic:

    dosage rate: 0.25 mg / lb
    concentration: 10 mg / ml
    weight of dog: 50 lbs.

    a. Dosage in mg: _____

    b. Dosage in ml: _____

2. Induce anesthesia in a 12 lb cat using 4% Surital at a dosage rate of 3 mg / lb

    a. How many mg are needed? _____

    b. How many ml are needed? _____

3. A 20 lb dog with a urinary tract infection will be treated with Gentomycin sulfate at the rate of 2 mg / lb twice a day for 5 days. The concentration of Gentomycin is 50 mg per ml. Determine:

    a. Dosage mg each treatment: _____

    b. Number of ml for each treatment: _____

    c. Total number of ml necessary for 5 days: _____

4. Tetracycline is dosed at 5 mg per lb every 8 hours.

    a. How many 250 mg capsules will a 50 pound dog need daily?

    b. How many capsules should be dispensed for 7 days of treatment?

5. Calculate the dosage in cc of sodium pentobarbital for each of the following rats if the rate is 5 mg per 100 g and the concentration: 64.8 mg per cc

    a. weight: 250 g   **b.** weight: 100 g

6. Calculate the dosage of sodium pentobarbital for a mouse if the rate is 60 mg / kg and sodium pentobarbital has 64.8 mg per cc. How many cc are needed if the weight of the mouse is

    a. 30 g   **b.** 45 g

7. Calculate the dosage of Vitamin C for a guinea pig. Rate: 2 mg/ 100 g B.W..; Vitamin C has 100 mg / ml. How many ml for each of the given weights of the guinea pigs?

    a. 0.550 kg   **b.** 620 g

Given the following information from a label, determine the necessary dosage(s):

8. Label information: Whipcide (Phthalofyne)
   Each ml contains 250 mg
   Sodium bicarbonate sufficient for pH adjustment
   Benzyl alcohol 0.01 ml
   Water for injection q.s.
   Usual dosage: 250 mg (1 ml) per kg

   How many cc (dosage) is needed for each of the following dogs:

   a. 45 lb **b.** 15 lb **c.** 22 lb **d.** 83 lb

9. Label information: Acepromozine
   Each ml contains 10 mg
   Usual dosage:
        Dogs: 0.25 mg up to 0.5 mg per lb B.W..
        Cats: 0.5 mg up to 1.0 mg per lb B.W..
        Horses: 2 g up to 4 g per 100 lb B.W..

   Determine the minimum dosage for each of the following:

   a. Dogs: How many cc for each animal?

   (i) 10 kg (ii) 14 kg (iii) 50 kg

188 Dosage and Concentration Applications

    b. Cats: How many cc for each animal?

        (i) 1.5 kg   (ii) 1 kg   (iii) 3.5 kg

    c. Horses: How many cc for each animal?

        (i) 500 kg   (ii) 350 kg   (iii) 900 kg

10. Label information: 5 mg/ml and 2 mg/kg. How many cc for each of the following dogs:

    a. 24 lbs.   **b.** 16 lbs.   **c.** 110 lbs.   **d.** $5\frac{1}{2}$ lbs.

Unit IV

Chapter 11
Diluting Concentrations and Infusion Rates

Diluting Solutions and Adjusting Concentrations

In a laboratory, solutions frequently are found in a concentrated form for ease of shipment and storage as well as economies of scale. The concentrated solution is called the *stock* solution. The concentration with which the solution is used can be less than this stock concentration. The result is that the technician must be able to dilute, usually with water, these stock solutions to the desired concentration for a particular use. This is accomplished by mixing some certain amount of stock solution with some amount of *diluent* to achieve the desired result.

For *example:* Isopropyl alcohol (rubbing alcohol) is shipped in concentrations of 100 %. alcohol. The most effective concentration against bacteria is 70%. The technician must mix the concentrated stock solution (100% alcohol) with water to reach the desired final concentration of 70%.

There are several techniques that can be used to determine the correct mix. We present the most widely used and most practical method. Remember that you *begin with a concentrated solution* and *always dilute* that solution to the desired concentration. A useful formula is provided:

Note: unless otherwise noted, the diluent is water.

$$C_1 \cdot V_1 = C_2 \cdot V_2$$

Infusion Rates and Diluting Solutions

C_1 is the original concentration of the stock solution

V_1 is the volume of the stock solution used

C_2 is the desired (final) concentration (the one you want to make)

V_2 is the volume of the final concentration

Examples: (i) You must prepare 4 L of a 70% isopropyl alcohol solution from the 100% stock solution. You must determine the volume of stock solution to use as well as the volume of the diluent, water, which must be mixed to achieve 4 liters of total volume.

$C_1 = 100\%$ $V_1 = ?$ determine the known information
$C_2 = 70\%$ $V_2 = 4 liters$

$C_1 \cdot V_1 = C_2 \cdot V_2$ use the formula

$100\% \times V_1 = 70\% \times 4 liters$ substitute the known information into the formula

$V_1 = \dfrac{70\% \times 4 liters}{100\%}$ cancel the percents; your answer will be in liters

$V_1 = \dfrac{280 L}{100}$

$V_1 = 2.8 L$ of 100% stock solution of isopropyl alcohol is needed

Now determine the volume of diluent (water) to add:

Total volume desired (final volume):   4.0 liters
Volume of (100%) alcohol: − 2.8 liters
Volume of water needed: 1.2 liters

(ii) You must prepare as much 40% solution isopropyl alcohol as possible from 2.3 L of 100% stock solution. Determine the volume of 40% solution that can be made and the volume of diluent, water, which is used to make the 40% solution.

$C_1 = 100\%$ $V_1 = 2.3$ L
$C_2 = 40\%$ $V_2 = ???$ Determine the known information

$$C_1 V_1 = C_2 V_2$$

$100\% \cdot 2.3\,L = 40\% \cdot V_2$ Use the formula and substitute the known
$V_2 = \dfrac{100\% \cdot 2.3\,L}{40\%}$ information. Simplify
$V_2 = 5.75\ Liters$

Total Volume	5.75 liters
Amount of 100% Alcohol	− 2.3 liters
Volume of water needed	3.45 liters

Practice Set XI – 1

Solve the following problems and determine the amount of diluent.

1. Isopropyl alcohol

stock	desired
$C_1 = 100\%$ $V_1 = ???$	$C_2 = 70\%$ $V_2 = 2.5$ L

Infusion Rates and Diluting Solutions

2. Ethyl alcohol

$C_1 = 95\%$ $V_1 = ???$
$C_2 = 70\%$ $V_2 = 3$ L

3. Formalin (recall that formalin is a liquid)

$C_1 = 10\%$ $V_1 = ???$
$C_2 = 2\%$ $V_2 = 12$ L

4. Acetic acid

$C_1 = 100\%$ $V_1 = 75$ ml
$C_2 = 2\%$ $V_2 = ???$

5. HCl (hydrochloric acid)

$C_1 = 100\%$ $V_1 = 20$ ml
$C_2 = 1\%$ $V_2 = ???$

6. NaHCO$_3$ (sodium bicarbonate)

$C_1 = 9\%$ $V_1 = ???$
$C_2 = 5\%$ $V_2 = 2500$ ml

7. Isopropyl alcohol

$C_1 = 100\%$ $V_1 = ???$
$C_2 = 70\%$ $V_2 = 3$ L

8. EtOH (ethyl alcohol)

$C_1 = 95\%$ $V_1 = ???$
$C_2 = 70\%$ $V_2 = 5$ L

9. NaOH (sodium hydroxide)

$C_1 = 30\%$ $V_1 = 700$ ml
$C_2 = 5\%$ $V_2 = ???$

10. Formalin

$C_1 = 100\%$ $V_1 = ???$
$C_2 = 10\%$ $V_2 = 30$ L

11. Formalin

$C_1 = 10\%$ $V_1 = ???$
$C_2 = 5\%$ $V_2 = 8$ L

Practice Set XI – 2

Solve each of the following. Determine the volume of stock solution needed *and* the volume of diluent.

1. Prepare 30 L of formalin from a 100% stock solution. How much formalin is needed to make:

   a. a 5% solution?   b. a 1% solution?

2. A stock solution of NaCl is 9%. Prepare 6 liters of a 0.9% saline solution. How much stock solution is needed?

3. Ethyl alcohol comes as a 95% stock solution. Prepare:

   a. 6 L of 90%   b. 9 l of 70%

4. Sodium hydroxide has been previously prepared in a concentration of 30% (C_1). But you need a concentration of 5% (C_2) and a volume of 1 L (1000 ml) (V_2). How many ml of the 30% solution will you have to use? How much water?

5. Isopropyl alcohol is 100% but the desired strength is 70%. How much of the 100% stock is needed to make 3 gallons of 70% solution?

6. If 20 L of alcohol (100%) was available, how many liters of 70% could you make?

7. 36% HCl needs to be diluted to 1%. Unfortunately there is only 200 ml of HCl left in the lab. How much will this make?

8. Prepare 25 L of a 10% formalin solution from a 100% stock solution. How much of the stock solution do you need? How much water will you use?

9. From the 10% formalin solution prepared in problem number **8**, make 30 L of: **a.** 5% solution and **b.** 1% solution. Determine the amount of 10% solution and the volume of water needed for each.

Practice Set XI – 3

Solve (You need not compute the amount of diluent.)

1. Isopropyl alcohol

    $C_1 = 100\%$ $C_2 = 70\%$
    $V_1 = ???$ $V_2 = 1$ L

2. Ethyl Alcohol

    $C_1 = 95\%$ $C_2 = 70\%$
    $V_1 = ???$ $V_2 = 4$ L

3. NaOH

    $C_1 = 30\%$ $C_2 = 5\%$
    $V_1 = 500$ ml $V_2 = ???$

4. Formalin

    $C_1 = 100\%$ $C_2 = 10\%$
    $V_1 = ???$ $V_2 = 20$ L

Infusion Rates and Diluting Solutions   199

5. Formalin

$C_1 = 10\%$ $C_2 = 5\%$
$V_1 = ???$ $V_2 = 5\ L$

6. Formalin

$C_1 = 10\%$ $C_2 = 2\%$
$V_1 = 1\ L$ $V_2 = ???$

7. Hydrogen peroxide

$C_1 = 100\%$ $C_2 = 2\%$
$V_1 = 50\ ml$ $V_2 = ???$

8. HCl

$C_1 = 100\%$ $C_2 = 1\%$
$V_1 = 10\ ml$ $V_2 = ???$

Practice Set XI – 4

$$C_1 \cdot V_1 = C_2 \cdot V_2$$

1. The isopropyl alcohol on hand is 100%, but the desired strength is 70%. How much of the 100% stock solution is needed to make 2 gallons of 70% solution?

2. 36% HCl needs to be diluted to 1%. There is 100 ml of HCl on hand. How much will this make?

3. Make 15 L of a 10% formalin solution from a 100% stock solution. How much of the stock solution is needed? How much water is needed?

4. From a 10% formalin solution, prepare 20 L of: **a.** 5%   **b.** 1%

5. Prepare 20 L of formalin for each of the following from a 100% stock solution,

    a. 5%   **b.** 1%

6. A stock solution of sodium chloride is 9%. From it, prepare 5 L of a 0.9% saline solution.

7. Ethyl alcohol comes in a 95% stock solution. Prepare:

    a. 5 L of 90%   **b.** 7 L of 70%

Infusion Rates

A dehydrated animal is re–hydrated according to generally accepted practices. Severely dehydrated animals – 10% or more dehydration, must be re–hydrated immediately. Within the first hour, fluids should be administered at the appropriate rate. In general, about half the necessary rehydration should occur within that first hour. More moderate dehydration, about 8% to 10% dehydration, can be re–hydrated during the first couple of hours of treatment. Less severe dehydration, up to about 8%, can be re–hydrated on a less immediate schedule.

The *infusion rate* is the rate at which a medication flows through a needle drip. Generally, there are two basic types of infusion rates, differing by the size of the needle bore used for delivery. Typically, the drip set is 15 drips per milliliter for animals over 20 pounds using a large bore needle and 60 drips per milliliter for animals under 20 pounds with a small bore.

We will examine two types of medication infusions. The first is fluid replacement therapy for dehydrated animals and the second is necessary hydration during the delivery of anesthesia during surgery. The two go hand–in–hand. Dehydrated animals must be rehydrated before surgery and animals that have surgery must have fluids that are lost during surgery replaced.

Example: (i) Determine the infusion rate for a 74 pound dog that is 5% dehydrated.

(a) Determine the total fluid volume. Multiply the percent dehydrated by the body weight in kilograms to get volume in liters. Convert to milliliters. Add to that result the daily maintenance fluid requirement, which is body weight in kilograms times 40 ml (a commonly accepted standard). The end result is the total fluid volume necessary for 24 hours.

replacement

$$\frac{74 \text{ lb} \mid 1 \text{ kg} \mid 0.05 \mid 1 \text{ L}}{2.2 \text{ lb} \mid \text{kg}} = 1.6818 \text{ Liters} = \underline{1682 \text{ ml}}$$

maintenance

$$\frac{74 \text{ lb} \mid 1 \text{ kg} \mid 40 \text{ ml}}{2.2 \text{ lb} \mid \text{kg}} = 1345 \text{ ml}$$

$$\underline{3027 \text{ ml}}$$

The total fluid volume, for replacement and maintenance, required for 24 hours is 3027 ml.

(b) Convert the total fluid necessary for 24 hours to milliliters per minute.

$$\frac{3027 \text{ ml}}{24 \text{ hrs}} \cdot \frac{1 \text{ hr}}{60 \text{ min}} \approx 2.1 \frac{ml}{min}$$

(c) Compute the drips per minute. Multiply the appropriate drip set times $^{ml}/_{min}$.

Drip sets: 15 $^{drips}/_{ml}$ for animals over 20 pounds

   60 $^{drips}/_{ml}$ for animals under 20 pounds

$$\frac{2.1 \text{ ml}}{min} \cdot \frac{15 \text{ drips}}{ml} = 31.5 \frac{drips}{min}$$

This is the necessary infusion rate for the 74 pound dog which was 5% dehydrated.

The second infusion rate computation involves a determination of the flow rate for hydrating during surgery. A common industry standard for this procedure is 4 ml/pound/hour. Use the body weight in pounds and dimensional analysis to convert to $^{ml}/_{min}$.

Example: We determine a 74 pound dog needs hydration at a rate of about 5 (4.9) $^{ml}/_{min}$

$$\frac{74 \text{ lb}}{1} \cdot \frac{4 \text{ ml}}{lb/hr} \cdot \frac{1 \text{ hr}}{60 \text{ min}} = 4.9 \, ^{ml}\!/_{min}$$

204   Infusion Rates and Diluting Solutions

Example: (ii) Determine the infusion rate for a 14 pound cat that is 8% dehydrated.

(computations follow)

(a) total fluid volume = 763.64

(b) ml/min = 0.5 ml/min

(c) drips/min = 30 drips/min

(d) anesthesia/surgery rate = 0.9 ml/min

(a) $$\frac{14 \text{ lb} \mid 1 \text{ kg} \mid .08 \mid 1 \text{ L} \mid 1000 \text{ ml}}{2.2 \text{ lb} \mid \mid 1 \text{ kg} \mid 1 \text{ L}} = 509.09 \text{ volume in ml}$$

$$\frac{14 \text{ lb} \mid 1 \text{ kg} \mid 40 \text{ ml}}{2.2 \text{ lb} \mid \text{kg}} = 254.55 \text{ maintenance volume in ml}$$

[add these for total daily volume of 763.64 ml]

(b) $$\frac{763.64 \text{ ml} \mid 1 \text{ hour}}{24 \text{ hrs} \mid 60 \text{ min}} = 0.5 \text{ ml/min}$$

(c) $$\frac{0.5 \text{ ml}}{\text{min}} \cdot \frac{60 \text{ drips}}{\text{ml}} = 30 \text{ drips}/\text{min}$$

(d) $$\frac{14 \text{ lb} \mid 4 \text{ ml} \mid 1 \text{ hr}}{ \mid \text{hr} \mid \text{lb} \mid 60 \text{ min}} = 0.9 \text{ ml}/\text{min}$$

Practice Set XI – 5

1. Determine the infusion rate for a 22 pound dog that is 6% dehydrated.

    a. total fluid volume _____

    b. ml/min _____

    c. drips/min _____

    d. anesthesia / surgery rate _____

2. Determine the infusion rate for a 450 lb horse that is 7% dehydrated.

    a. total fluid volume _____

    b. ml/min _____

    c. drips/min _____

    d. anesthesia / surgery rate _____

3. Determine the infusion rate for a 6 lb kitten that is 6% dehydrated.

    a. total fluid volume _____

    b. ml/min _____

    c. drips/min _____

    d. anesthesia / surgery rate _____

4. Determine the infusion rate for a 68 pound dog that is 4% dehydrated.

    a. total fluid volume _____

    b. ml/min _____

    c. drips/min _____

    d. anesthesia / surgery rate _____

5. Determine the infusion rate for a 46 lb Collie that is 6% dehydrated.

    a. total fluid volume _____

    b. ml/min _____

    c. drips/min _____

    d. anesthesia / surgery rate _____

6. Determine the infusion rate for a 14 lb animal that is 8% dehydrated.

    a. total fluid volume _____

    b. ml/min _____

    c. drips/min _____

    d. anesthesia / surgery rate _____

7. Determine the infusion rate for a 105 lb Chow that is 4% dehydrated.

   a. total fluid volume _____

   b. ml/min _____

   c. drips/min _____

   d. anesthesia / surgery rate _____

8. Determine the infusion rate for a 147 lb Chimp that is 5% dehydrated.

   a. total fluid volume _____

   b. ml/min _____

   c. drips/min _____

   d. anesthesia / surgery rate _____

9. Determine the infusion rate for a 1300 horse that is 6% dehydrated.

   a. total fluid volume _____

   b. ml/min _____

   c. drips/min _____

   d. anesthesia / surgery rate _____

10. Determine the infusion rate for a 8 lb cat that is 4% dehydrated.

    a. total fluid volume _____

    b. ml/min _____

    c. drips/min _____

    d. anesthesia / surgery rate _____

Chapter 12
Graphs and Graphing Techniques

A graph is a visual means of presenting numerical data to show relationships between one set of numbers and another. Graphs of data sometimes must be prepared by the technician. Usually the graph will have a vertical axis called the y axis (ordinate) and a horizontal axis called the x axis (abscissa).

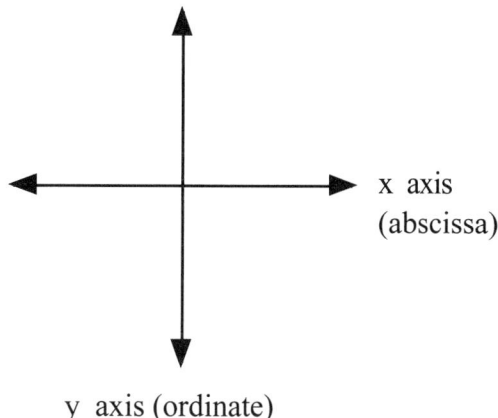

x axis (abscissa)

y axis (ordinate)

Each axis is divided into the desired units. These units describe some term of the experiment which can be measured. An example might be light absorbed measured on one axis and concentration of a solution measured on the other axis. Heart rate, respiration, or pulse over time might be another example, as well as animal weight versus age or height.

Plotting the graph

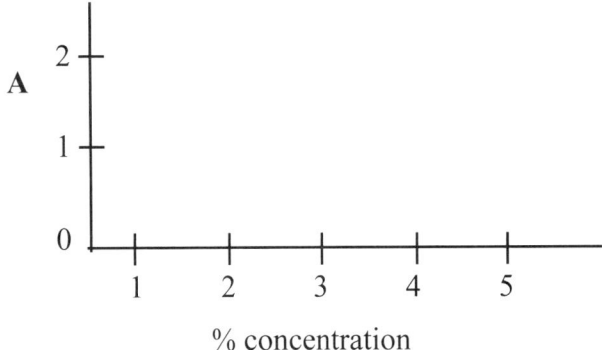

Generally, it makes no difference which item of interest is plotted on the x-axis and which is plotted on the y-axis. The divisions are spaced and numbered according to a convenient measurement. In the example shown, (Fig. 12.1) time is measured in minutes and temperature in degrees Celsius. The time scale could have been shown in seconds but the graph would have been larger (much more "spread out"). In this case, the time measurement is on the x-axis and temperature scale is on the y-axis.

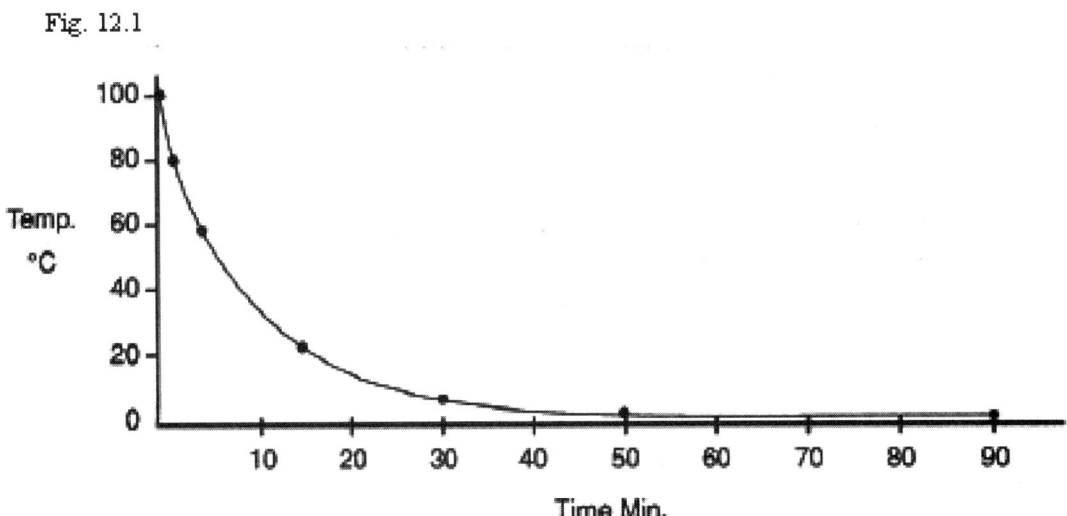

The numbers for the upper limit should be equal to or slightly larger than the largest data value. You would not select 80 minutes when the last point turned out to be at 90 minutes since this would eliminate some of the data. The lower limit, likewise, must be less than or equal to the lowest value. In many cases the lowest value is zero. But be aware of distorted (truncated) graphs which do not start at zero. However, many legitimate graphs do start at some number other than zero.

Some *examples* of graphs used in Veterinary Medical Technology:

(i) **ECG** graphs – top view indicates interference occurred during the recording. The bottom view is a standard result.

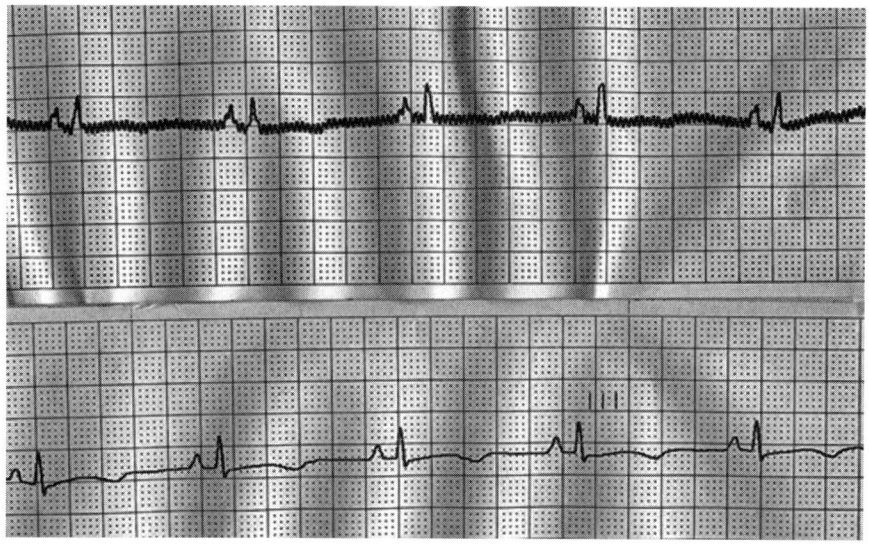

(ii)   Chart showing respiration rate and pulse rate.

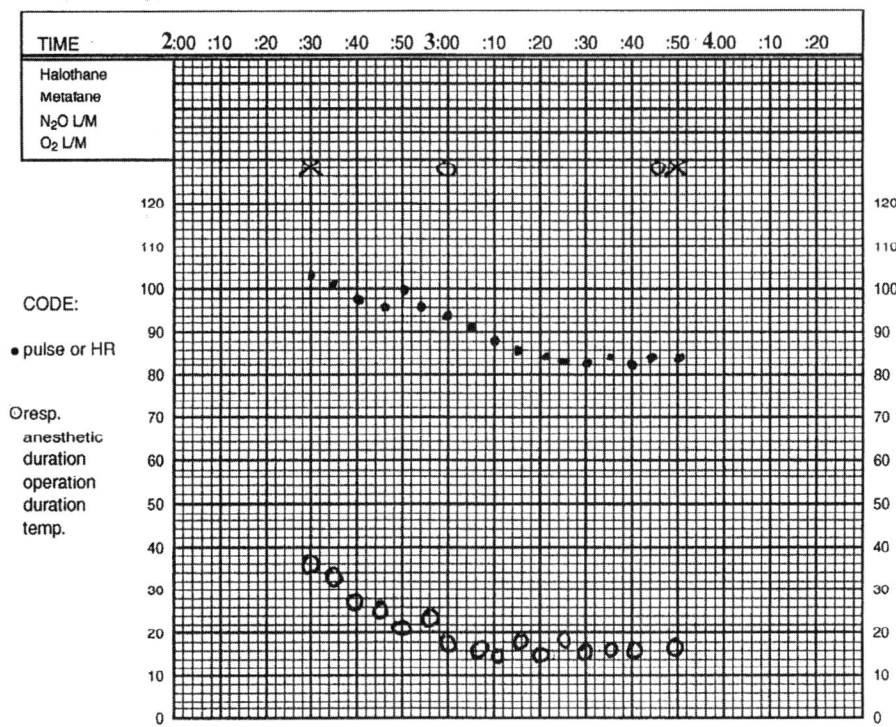

(iii)   Blood and Urine chemistries are usually line graphs.

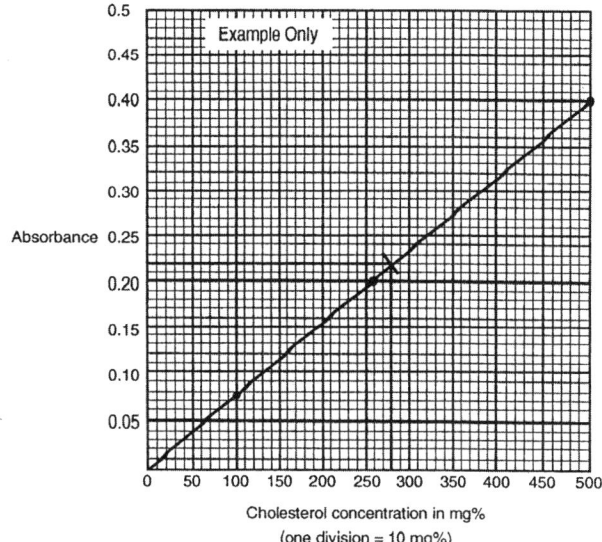

Plotting data on the graph can show changes, trends, and relative quantities.

The x-axis is designated one variable (time, in this example) while the vertical y-axis is designated as another variable (heart rate).

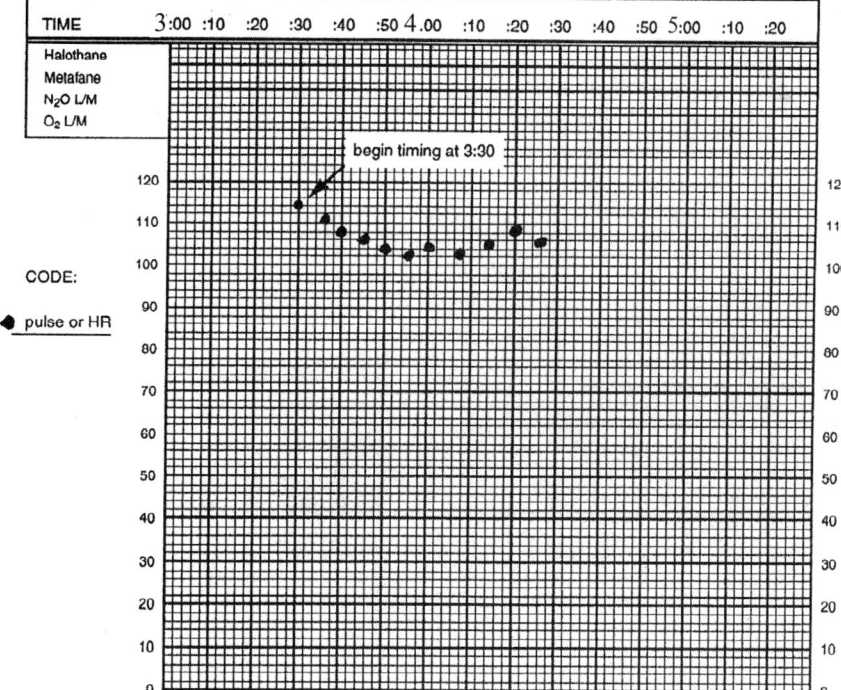

It is common to label each axis with the type of measurement such as time, rate and temperature and also with the respective units (sec, min, beats per min, degrees C.)

214   Graphs and Graphing Techniques

A two dimensional rectangular graph has four quadrants. The center point is called the origin and is labeled (0, 0). Any point in the plane, that is, on the graph is denoted with an *ordered* pair of numbers (x, y) which tell the location of that particular point. It is called an ordered pair since the order matters. The first number denotes movement left and right in line with the x–axis; the second number gives the vertical movement.

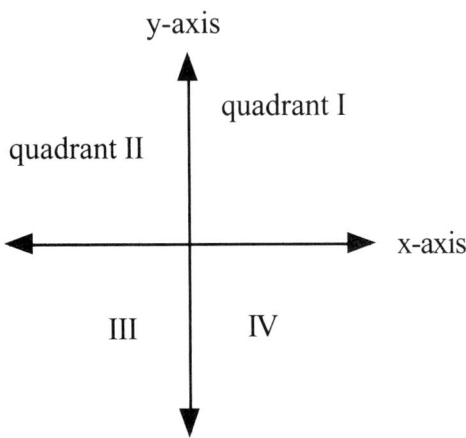

The most common uses of graphs for the veterinary technician involves quadrant I or quadrants I and IV

Examples:

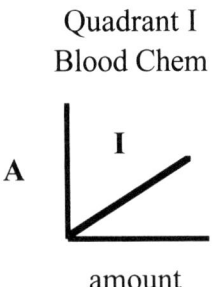

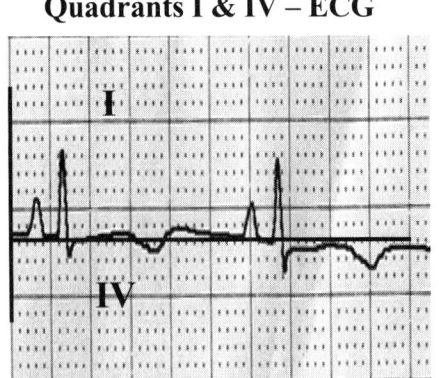

Plotting rectangular coordinates

Plotting in quadrant I. (The most common case)

Both coordinates will be positive.

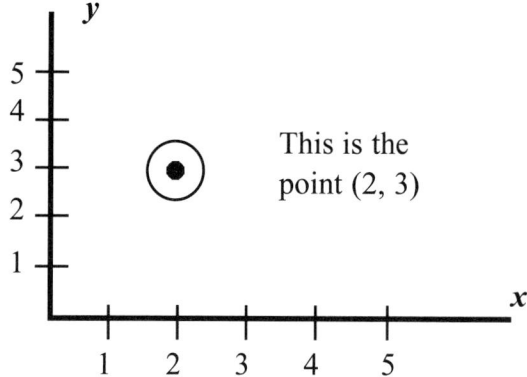

The first value in the ordered pair (2) denotes the distance in line with the *x*–axis; the second value of the ordered pair (3) denotes the distance vertically in line with the *y*–axis. The point is plotted where the two corresponding imaginary lines meet.

An example best illustrates how to determine where points on graphs should be placed. In this example, use 0.30 A, which is a measure of the quantity of light absorbed and a concentration of the solution of 3%.

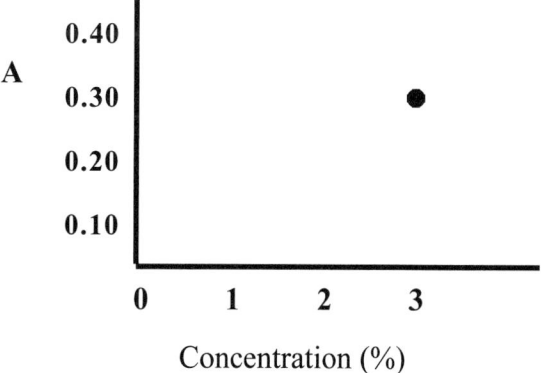

Start at zero (0) and proceeds 3 units to the right along the x-axis. This corresponds to the 3% concentrate. Next, proceed vertically for 3 units which corresponds to .30 on the scale of the y-axis. At this point, make a dot (as shown.) The procedure could have been reversed with no effect on the results. Going up 3 units and then over 3 units will yield the same point on the graph.

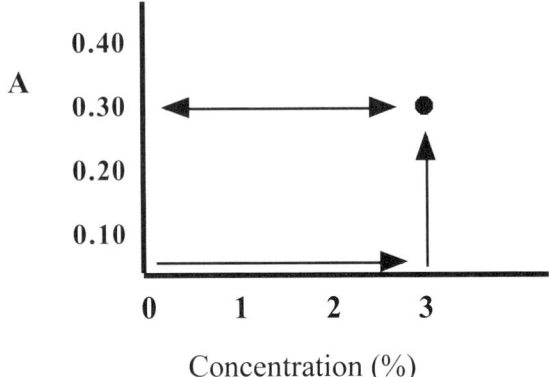

Other known or observed values may be plotted on the same graph. As in the graph example above, the following points are plotted in the same manner. Those points are joined with a straight line.

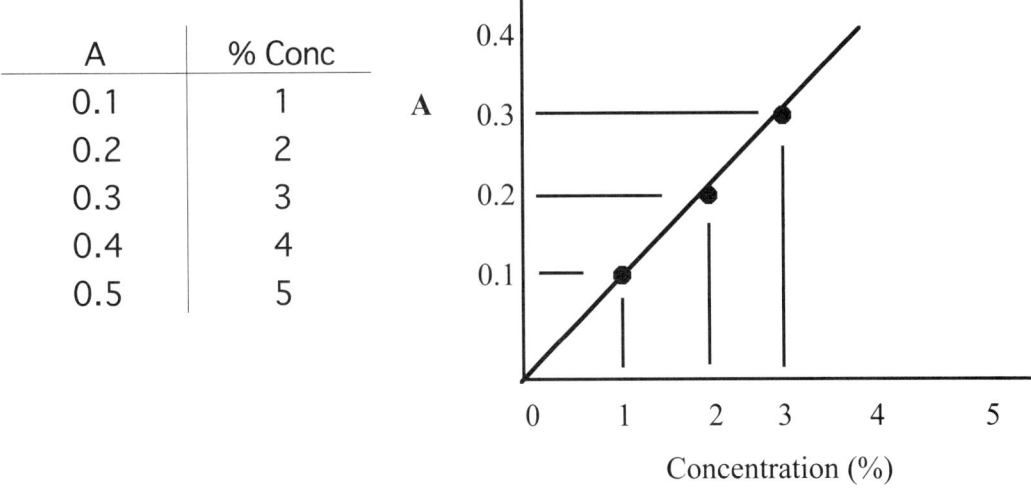

A	% Conc
0.1	1
0.2	2
0.3	3
0.4	4
0.5	5

Plotting a Standard Curve (or Standard Plot)

Although referred to as a standard curve it is actually a straight line. It is composed of points derived from known values on both the x- and y-axes.

Many chemical solutions have known concentrations. The absorbency of light, A, is determined using a spectrophotometer. These values can then be plotted on a graph.

Example: Using the given information, plot a standard curve of concentration at absorbency (A).

Concentration v Absorbency

Conc (%)	A
1	0.05
2	0.10
3	0.15
4	0.20
5	0.25

Determining values from an unknown:

Once a standard curve has been plotted, it can be used to determine concentrations of other solutions by measuring Absorbency using a spectrophotometer.

Using the standard curve, the concentration of an unknown solution is placed in a spectrophotometer and the absorbency is determined. On the graph shown below, (1) go up the y-axis (A) until that value is reached. (2) Then proceed parallel to the x-axis (concentration) until the standard curve is intersected. (3) Now drop vertically to the x-axis to (4) read the corresponding concentration of the solution.

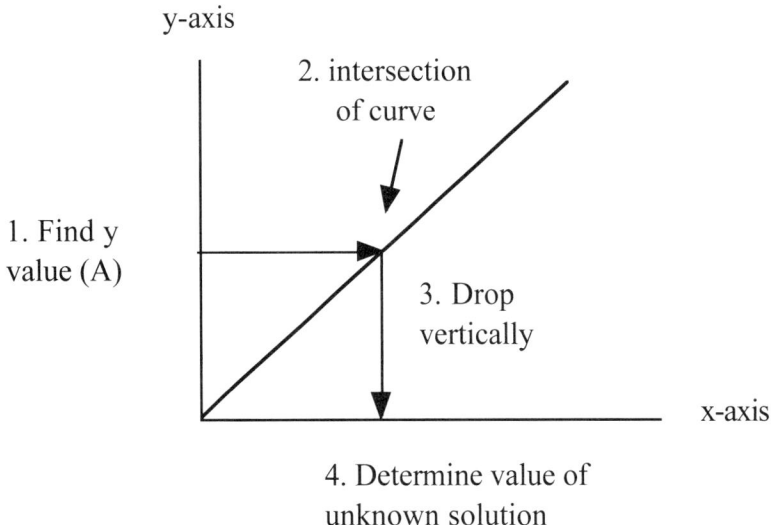

Practice Set XII – 1

1. Using the given chart of concentration *v* Absorbency (A), plot the points, draw a standard curve and determine the concentrations for the given absorbencies to complete the table that follows.

A	Concentration (mg%)
0.09	100
0.23	260
0.45	500

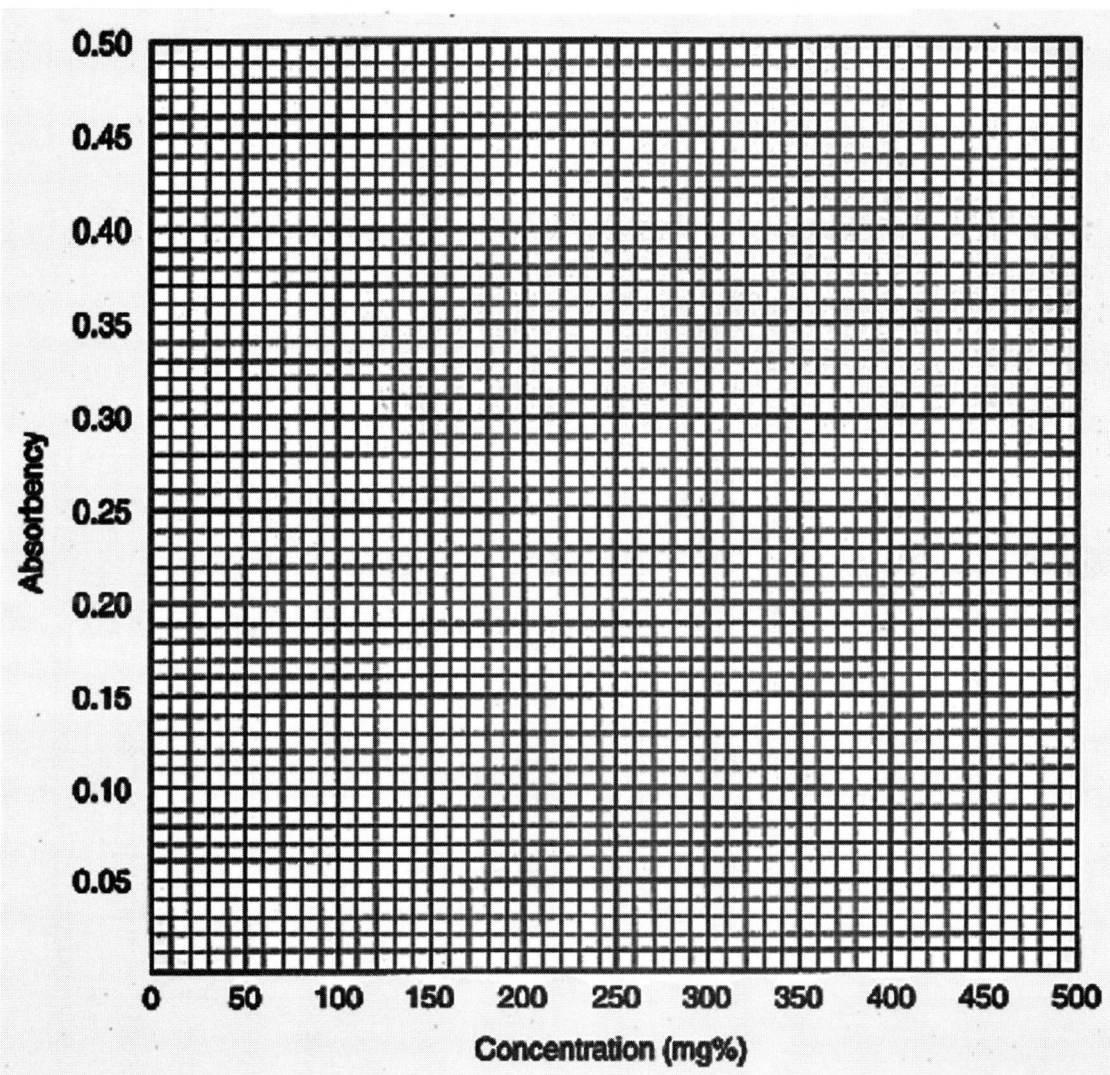

Unknown Solution	A	Concentration
A	0.16	_____
B	0.22	_____
C	0.15	_____
D	0.09	_____
E	0.12	_____
F	0.24	_____

2. Given the following graph and values, interpolate for cholesterol levels to complete the chart that follows.

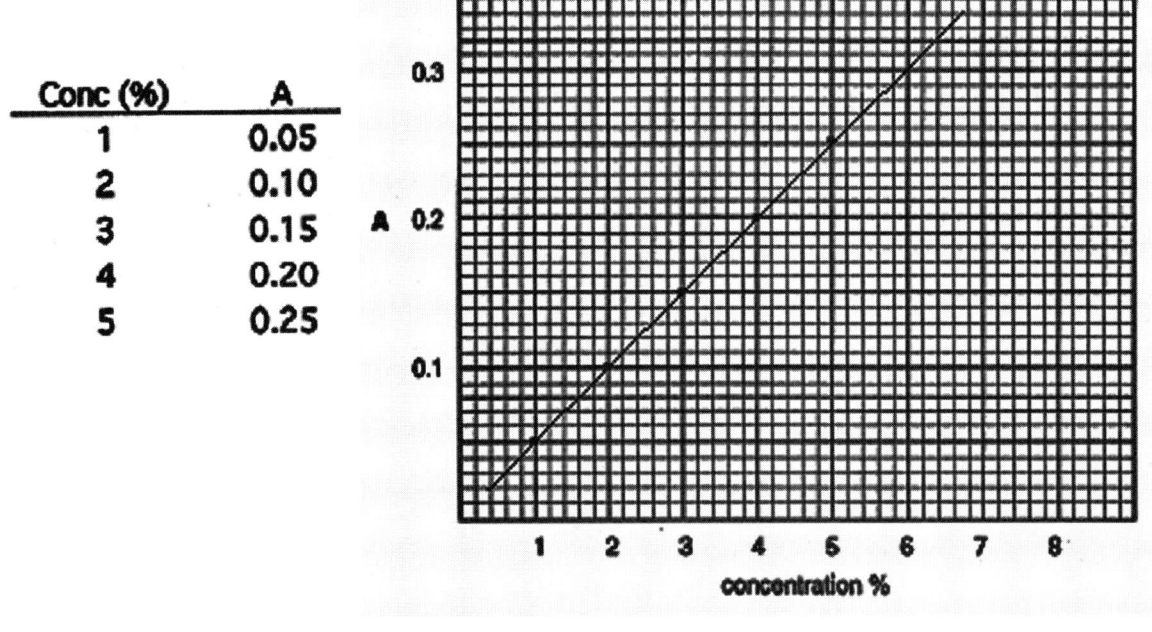

Conc (%)	A
1	0.05
2	0.10
3	0.15
4	0.20
5	0.25

Sample	Absorbency	concentration %
A	0.10	_____
B	0.20	_____
C	0.30	_____
D	0.35	_____
E	0.27	_____
F	0.18	_____

Plotting graphs using quadrants I and IV such as for an EKG.

All values along the x-axis are positive. However, y values may be positive or negative. Those y values that lie above the x-axis are positive (in quadrant I) and those below the x-axis (in quadrant IV) are negative.

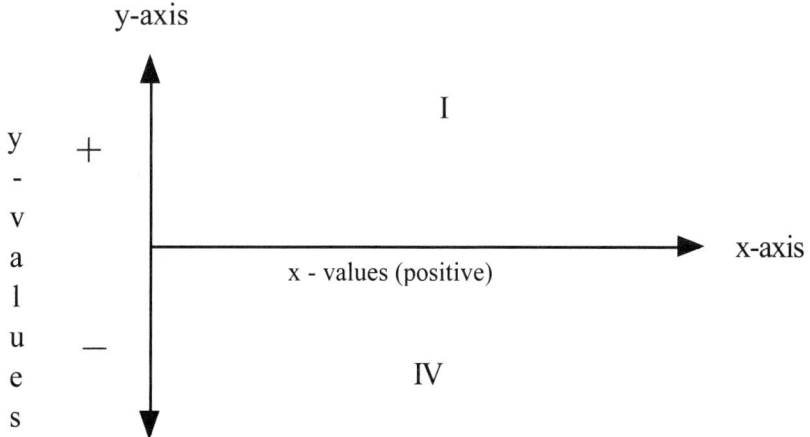

3. Recall that coordinates for a point are given as an ordered pair, (x, y). On the following graph, find the (x, y) ordered pair values for each lettered point on the graph.

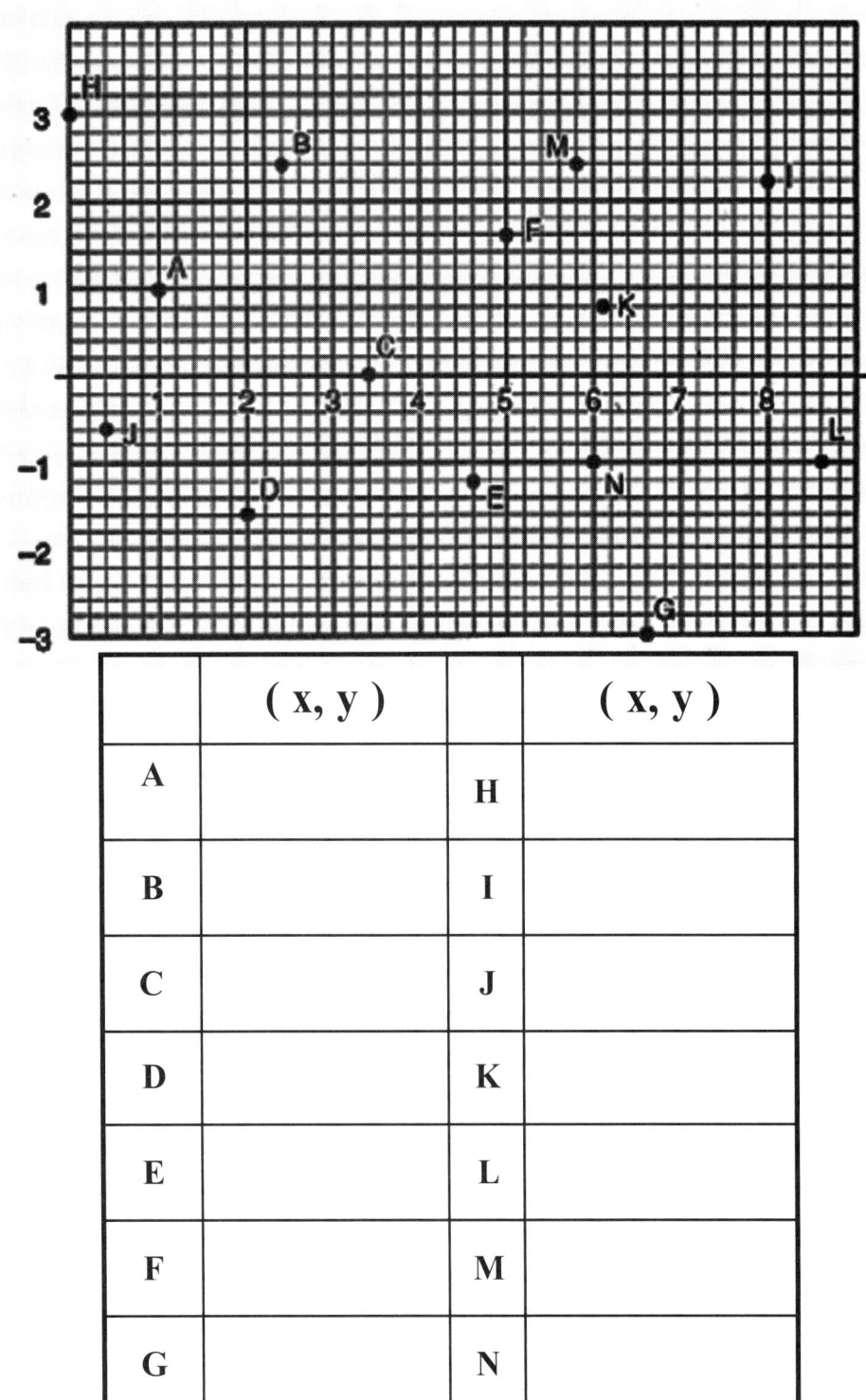

	(x, y)		(x, y)
A	(1, 1)	H	(0, 3)
B	(2.5, 2.5)	I	(8.5, 2.5)
C	(3, 0.25)	J	(−0.5, −0.5)
D	(2, −1.5)	K	(6, 1)
E	(4.5, −1)	L	(8.5, −0.5)
F	(5, 1.75)	M	(5.5, 2.5)
G	(7, −3)	N	(6, −1)

4. The following graph is an example of an ECG recording. Assume 1 cm = 1 MV on the y-axis and 2.5 cm = 1 sec along the x-axis. Determine the millivolt at several positions as indicated by each letter and how much time has elapsed at each letter. The vertical line on the left is 0 seconds.

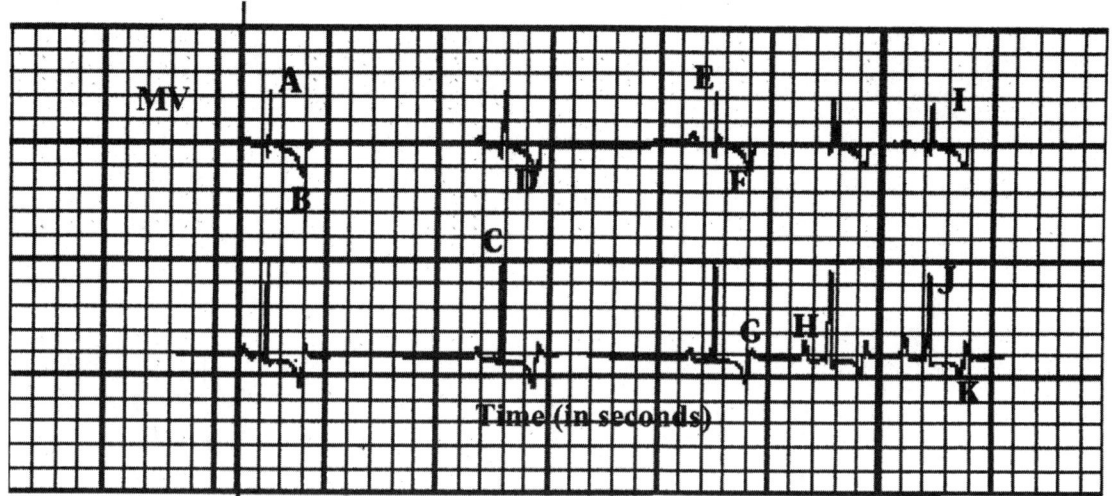

Letter	Time	Millivolt
A	_____	_____
B	_____	_____
C	_____	_____
D	_____	_____
E	_____	_____
F	_____	_____
G	_____	_____
H	_____	_____
I	_____	_____
J	_____	_____
K	_____	_____

Unit V

Chapter 13
Statistics

In every technical occupation, an understanding of basic statistical concepts is essential. In this section, we explore some of the common statistical concepts, terms, numerical methods, and techniques that will form a basis for understanding. This is meant as an overview and in no way can this one chapter alone provide the technician with the skills they will surely need in a laboratory or clinical setting. A semester course in basic statistics is strongly recommended.

Knowledge of statistics allows you to make educated, informed decisions based upon data (information). Statistics is the study of collecting, organizing, and interpreting numerical information and making decisions based upon that information. Knowledge of statistics can help one make decisions about kennel occupancy rates, staffing issues, inventory and payroll.

In this chapter, the concepts of measures of central tendency and measures of variation will be explored.

In statistics there are three common "averages". The *mean*, denoted $\bar{x}$ (x–bar), which is the "average" most people think of when they think of the term average. The mean is arrived at by adding all the relevant items and dividing by how many of those items there are.

Example: Determine the mean of the following values. 85, 90, 92, 95, 94

$$\frac{85 + 90 + 92 + 95 + 94}{5} = 91.2 \qquad \text{The mean is 91.2}$$

Another type of average is called the *median*. Often, this number is more meaningful than the mean. The median is the middle number of a set of data that has been put in order from least to greatest. For the number set above, 85, 90, (92) 94, 95 . The median is 92. If the number of data values is even, then the median is the mean of the two middle values.

A third type of average is called the *mode*. The mode is the number that occurs most often in a set of data. For the previous values: 85, 90, 92, 94, 95, there is no number that occurs more than any other, therefore, there is no mode. For the values: 2, 3, 4, 4, 4, 5, 6, 6, 8, the mode is 4, since there are more representations of the value 4 than any other value.

These averages, called *measures of central tendency* describe some central point or measure of the data and indicate how data is grouped.

Measures of variation, on the other hand, describe how data is spread out. The *range* is a measure of the difference between the highest data value and the lowest. The measures of *variation* and *standard deviation* tell how much data varies around some middle value.

These measures of variation can describe if the data is all closely grouped or spread widely apart. *Standard deviation* is the square root of the *variance*. Many modern calculators perform these statistical functions making it easy to grasp the importance of the data rather than distracting you with tedious computations.

All fields have their own language and notation. Statistics is no different. Some notation typically found in the study of statistics include:

n used for the number of data values

$\bar{x}$ read as x-bar; symbolizes the mean

$\tilde{x}$ read as x-tilde; symbolizes the median

s^2 symbolizes the variance of a sample

s standard deviation; $s = \sqrt{s^2}$ means standard deviation = $\sqrt{\text{variance}}$

Σ sigma (uppercase); summation = "to sum"

Summation notation is used in many statistical formulas. It is a notational device indicating addition and tells the user what should be added and the conditions for the addition.

These are called index numbers; the lower tells where to begin (in this case with the first data value) and the upper tells where to stop (the nth value)

$$\sum_{i=1}^{n} x_i$$

This part tells what is being added and what to do with it; do this part first, then add all the resultant values

In statistics, the index numbers are usually omitted since *all* the data values are used.

Examples: (i) Given the data: {2, 3, 6, 7, 9, 9}; Determine $\sum x$

This notation tells us to take each value in the data set, and then add, or sum, the result.

$$\sum x = 2 + 3 + 6 + 7 + 9 + 9 = 36$$

(ii) Given {2, 3, 6, 7, 9, 9}; Determine $\sum x^2$

$$\sum x^2 = 2^2 + 3^2 + 6^2 + 7^2 + 9^2 + 9^2 = 260$$

Note: in this case, first square each value, **then** add.

(iii) Given {2, 3, 6, 7, 9, 9}; Determine $\left(\sum x\right)^2$

$$\left(\sum x\right)^2 = (2 + 3 + 6 + 7 + 9 + 9)^2 = (36)^2 = 1296$$

Note the difference. In this case, the notation tells us to add the values **first**, then square the result.

Pay particular attention to the distinction between the second and third examples!

Practice Set XIII – 1

Given the set of numbers {4, 8, 9, 2, 5}, Compute.

1. $\sum x$

2. $\dfrac{\sum x}{n}$

3. $\sum x^2$

4. $\sum (x - 5.6)$

5. $\sum (x - 5.6)^2$

Given the values $x_1 = 12$, $x_2 = 11$, $x_3 = 14$, $x_4 = 13$, Compute.

6. $\sum x$

7. $\sum x^2$

8. $\sum (x - 1)^2$

Now that you have had a little practice with using summation notation, we are going to introduce some formulas to use in computing statistics. Recall the mean, $\bar{x} = \dfrac{\Sigma x}{n}$, is the typical average which is the sum of all the data values divided by the number of pieces of data. The median, $\tilde{x}$, is the middle value of the ordered set of data. The mode is the data value that occurs more than any other number. If there is no such number, there is no mode. The range is the difference between the highest and lowest values. The variance, s^2, which is one measure of how data varies, is determined by the computational formula, variance $= \dfrac{n\Sigma x^2 - (\Sigma x)^2}{n(n-1)}$. The standard deviation, s, is the square root of the variance, $s = \sqrt{\text{variance}}$. We'll begin with a set of data, say test scores, and explore several important statistical concepts along the way.

Example: On 24 randomly chosen days, the number of patients was recorded. Determine the mean, median, mode, range, variance and standard deviation for the data.

| 66 | 79 | 53 | 65 | 89 | 76 | 73 | 84 | 76 | 69 | 77 | 97 |
| 75 | 78 | 80 | 71 | 86 | 68 | 64 | 76 | 86 | 72 | 76 | 68 |

Order the scores from the smallest value to the largest. This is necessary to find the median.

53	69	76	80
64	71	76	84
65	72	76	86
66	73	77	86
68	75	78	89
68	76	79	97

With statistical problems, it is often helpful to organize the data in tables or columns. Since we need to know the sum of all the x and the sum of each of the x squared …

x	x^2	
53	2809	
64	4096	
65	4225	
66	4356	
68	4624	
68	4624	
69	4761	
71	5041	
72	5184	
73	5329	
75	5625	
76	5776	
76	5776	
76	5776	
76	5776	
77	5929	
78	6084	
79	6241	
80	6400	
84	7056	
86	7396	
86	7396	
89	7921	
97	9409	
1804	137610	*Totals*

The number of data values, $n = 24$. The mean, $\bar{x} = \dfrac{\sum x}{n}$, $\dfrac{1804}{24} = 75.2$.

The median is the mean of the two middle numbers – the first and second values of 76 are the middle numbers – their average is 76, so the median is 76.

The mode, the number that occurs most often is 76.

The range, the difference between the highest and lowest values, is 44 ($97 - 53 = 44$).

The variance, found by formula, $\text{variance} = \dfrac{n\sum x^2 - (\sum x)^2}{n(n-1)}$

$= \dfrac{(24)(137{,}610) - (1804)^2}{24(24-1)}$

$= \dfrac{3302640 - 3254416}{24 \times 23}$

$= \dfrac{48224}{552}$

$= 87.36$ variance

The substitutions for $n = 24$, the sum of the x's squared $= 137610$ and the sum of the x values $= 1804$. Simplify.

The standard deviation is the square root of the variance, $\sqrt{87.36} = 9.35$.

A quick and easy way to organize and present data is to use a *stem–and–leaf diagram*.

A stem-and-leaf diagram has *stems* on the left of the vertical bar and *leaves* on the right. Since the data are all two-digits, the stems are the tens place while the units will be the leaves.

```
Key:  5 | 3 = 53

5 | 3
6 | 4 5 6 8 8 9
7 | 1 2 3 5 6 6 6 6 7 8 9
8 | 0 4 6 6 9
9 | 7
```

This diagram preserves all the original data and is easy to complete. On the other hand, it is not very useful for very large data sets.

Practice Set XIII – 2

    Circle the correct response: **T – True   F – False**

1. For the data set: 5, 9, 12, 11, 2, 4, 9, and 8, the range would be 10.   T   F

2. For the sample: 1, 8, 7, 2, 9, 15, and 18, the mean is 7.6.   T   F

3. For the sample: 19, 21, 19, 17, 18, 19, and 21, the mode is 19.   T   F

4. For the sample: 1.3, 2.7, 8.9, 7.3, 9.2, and 8.1, the median is 8.9.   T   F

    Multiple Choice: Circle the letter of the correct response

5. Measures of central tendency are quantities which:

    (a) numerically describe data.   (b) describe the distribution of data.

    (c) describe the grouping of data.   (d) describe qualitative data.

6. Measures that describe how the data is distributed or spread out are:

    (a) range.   (b) variance.

    (c) standard deviation.   (d) all of the above.

7. Calculate the range and standard deviation (listed in that order) of the following sample test grades:

    87   75   68   57   69   78

    (a) 30, 9.3   (b) 30, 10.19   (c) 25, 9.3   (d) 25, 10.19

Practice Set XIII – 3

1. Determine the mean and standard deviation for the temperatures taken from 10 healthy dogs.

100°F	101.7°F	99.9°F	103.2°F	102.4°F
100.5°F	102°F	104.5°F	102.8°F	103.5°F

2. Kennel occupancy rates often dictate how easy it might be to reserve a space at the last minute and determine the average cost of that space. Kennel spaces are often discounted in areas with low occupancy. Occupancy rates for kennels in a major city are given below.

56	89	79	71	70	60	60	61	62	63	64	65
81	73	68	72	56	59	60	62	73	64	72	67

    a. Make a stem-and-leaf plot for the given data.

    b. Determine the mean, median and mode.

    c. Find the range and standard deviation.

3. According to *The Merck Veterinary Manual*, the standard weight of a young colt is about 60 kilograms. Determine the mean, median and mode of the weights of colts treated in a certain practice. Also find the range, variance and standard deviation. Weights given in kg.

      58   60   62   64   61   56   62   62   54   64

4. There is concern about staff turnover in a particular practice. A survey was conducted and the number of months that staff was on the job was recorded. Find the mean, median, mode, range and standard deviation that employees have been on the job.

      10   2   40   15   27   6   9   8   4   25   30
      38   14   5   12   18   20   35   44   7   24   9

238   Statistics

The *weighted average* is a measure of the mean which assigns certain "weights" to different measures. For example, in a particular class papers may account for 20% of your grade, quizzes for 30%, tests for 40%, attendance for 10%. Your grade for each item is affected by the weight of that item. The formula, $\bar{x}_w = \dfrac{\sum xw}{\sum w}$, uses each x multiplied by its weight and the result summed, then divided by the sum of the weights.

Example: Sally and Bill were in the same English class. Sally had grade averages of 90 for papers, 89 for tests, 95 for quizzes and 100 for attendance. Bill had grade averages of 84 for papers, 93 for tests, 86 for quizzes and 85 for attendance. Determine the weighted average of each student.

$$\dfrac{90(.20) + 89(.40) + 95(.30) + 100(.10)}{.20 + .30 + .40 + .10} =$$

Add the grades multiplied by their corresponding weights

Add the weights

$$\dfrac{18 + 35.6 + 28.5 + 10}{1} = 92.1$$

Simplify. Sally's grade is a 92

$$\dfrac{84(.20) + 93(.40) + 86(.30) + 85(.10)}{.20 + .30 + .40 + .10} =$$

Add the grades multiplied by their corresponding weights

Add the weights

$$\dfrac{16.8 + 37.2 + 25.8 + 8.5}{1} = 88.3$$

Simplify. Bill's grade is an 88

5. A pay scale is determined by scores given to an employee by their supervisor for such things as accurate records, good work habits, attitude dealing with customers and ability to get along with fellow employees. Weights are assigned as follows: 2 for attendance and good work habits, 3 for record keeping, 4 for customer relations and 2 for interaction with coworkers. What would be an employee's weighted average if her scores were, on a scale from 1 to 10, 9 for attendance, 8 for keeping accurate records, 8 for customer relations, and 6 for getting on with coworkers.

Selected Solutions

Chapter 1
Practice Set I – 1

1. 20 **3.** 64 **5.** 99 **7.** 448 **9.** 3333 **11.** 4 **13.** 3 **15.** 57 **17.** 32 **19.** MCMLXXIII

21. IX **23.** XXIX **25.** XLIX **27.** MMCCXXII **29.** IV **31.** LIV **33.** LXXVI

Chapter 2
Practice Set II - 1

1. a. $\frac{2}{4} = \frac{1}{2}$ **b.** $\frac{3}{8}$ **c.** $\frac{5}{9}$ **d.** $\frac{5}{12}$ **3. a.** $\frac{1}{36}$ yard **b.** $\frac{35}{36}$ yd **c.** $\frac{13}{36}$ yd **d.** $\frac{19}{36}$ yd

5. a. $\$\frac{12}{100} = \$\frac{3}{25}$ **b.** $\$\frac{37}{100}$ **c.** $\$\frac{50}{100} = \$\frac{1}{2}$ **d.** $\$\frac{99}{100}$

Practice Set II-2

1. $\frac{3}{5}$ **3.** $\frac{1}{2}$ **5.** 4 **7.** $\frac{1}{2}$ **9.** $\frac{8}{9}$ **11.** $\frac{5}{9}$

Practice Set II - 3

1. $3\frac{1}{3}$ **3.** $6\frac{1}{4}$ **5.** $2\frac{3}{16}$ **7.** $\frac{13}{3}$ **9.** $\frac{19}{10}$ **11.** $\frac{35}{9}$

Practice Set II - 4

1. a. $\frac{1}{4}$ **b.** $\frac{1}{6}$ **c.** $\frac{24}{25}$ **d.** $\frac{1}{4}$ **e.** $\frac{1}{2}$ **f.** $\frac{1}{6}$ **g.** $\frac{1}{8}$ **h.** $\frac{1}{9}$

3. a. 3 **b.** $6\frac{6}{7}$ **c.** $6\frac{1}{9}$ **d.** $7\frac{1}{9}$ **e.** $21\frac{1}{4}$ **f.** $3\frac{4}{7}$ **g.** $4\frac{1}{5}$ **h.** $5\frac{1}{4}$

Chapter 3
Practice Set III – 1

1. $\frac{4}{3} = 1\frac{1}{3}$ **3.** $\frac{7}{2} = 3\frac{1}{2}$ **5.** $\frac{20}{7} = 2\frac{6}{7}$ **7.** $\frac{5}{3} = 1\frac{2}{3}$

Practice Set III – 2

1. $\frac{1}{9}$ **3.** $\frac{1}{12}$ **5.** $\frac{6}{20} = \frac{3}{10}$ **7.** $\frac{15}{32}$

Selected Solutions

Practice Set III – 3

1. $\dfrac{4}{15}$ 3. $\dfrac{3}{20}$ 5. $\dfrac{3}{5}$ 7. $\dfrac{1}{4}$ 9. $\dfrac{1}{6}$ 11. $\dfrac{2}{5}$

Practice Set III – 4

1. 32 3. 22 5. $13\dfrac{1}{5}$ 7. $9\dfrac{1}{3}$ 9. $9\dfrac{4}{5}$ 11. $56\dfrac{1}{4}$ 13. $8\dfrac{5}{16}$

Practice Set III – 5

1. $41\dfrac{1}{4}$ 3. 21 pounds

Practice Set III – 6

1. $\dfrac{5}{6}$ 3. $1\dfrac{1}{5}$ 5. $\dfrac{5}{9}$ 7. $2\dfrac{1}{10}$ 9. 48

Practice Set III – 7

1. 15 3. 16 5. 24 7. 64 9. 70

Practice Set III – 8

1. $\dfrac{7}{40}$ 3. $\dfrac{1}{16}$ 5. $\dfrac{3}{11}$

Practice Set III – 9

1. $26\dfrac{2}{3}$ 3. $\dfrac{13}{30}$ 5. $\dfrac{1}{4}$ 7. 18 9. $1\dfrac{1}{5}$

Practice Set III – 10

1. $\dfrac{7}{9}$ 3. $\dfrac{2}{5}$ 5. $\dfrac{1}{2}$ 7. $\dfrac{1}{6}$ 9. $1\dfrac{1}{2}$ 11. $1\dfrac{1}{2}$
13. $5\dfrac{1}{3}$ 15. 12 17. 8 19. 16 21. 24 23. $\dfrac{1}{4}$
25. $\dfrac{10}{29}$ 27. 8 29. $\dfrac{8}{25}$ 31. 6

Chapter 4
Practice Set IV – 1

1. $\dfrac{7}{8}$ 3. $\dfrac{4}{5}$ 5. $\dfrac{3}{7}$ 7. $\dfrac{5}{4} = 1\dfrac{1}{4}$

Practice Set IV – 2

1. $\dfrac{1}{3}$ 3. $\dfrac{2}{3}$ 5. $\dfrac{2}{3}$ 7. $\dfrac{5}{8}$ 9. $\dfrac{3}{8}$ 11. $\dfrac{9}{14}$
13. $\dfrac{1}{3}$ 15. $1\dfrac{5}{8}$

Practice Set IV – 3

1. $13\dfrac{5}{12}$ 3. $19\dfrac{5}{8}$ 5. $15\dfrac{3}{4}$ 7. $22\dfrac{3}{5}$ 9. $13\dfrac{1}{2}$ 11. $15\dfrac{1}{2}$
13. $16\dfrac{1}{2}$ 15. $8\dfrac{7}{9}$

Practice Set IV – 4

1. $3\dfrac{11}{16}$ 3. $4\dfrac{17}{20}$

Practice Set IV – 5

1. $3\dfrac{11}{12}$ 3. $8\dfrac{2}{3}$

Practice Set IV – 6

1. $\dfrac{1}{3}$ 3. $\dfrac{7}{11}$

Practice Set IV – 7

1. $\dfrac{3}{8}$ 3. $\dfrac{1}{6}$ 5. $\dfrac{7}{32}$ 7. $\dfrac{7}{20}$ 9. $\dfrac{3}{5}$ 11. 1

Practice Set IV – 8

1. $3\frac{3}{8}$ 3. $4\frac{1}{4}$ 5. $1\frac{1}{6}$ 7. $9\frac{1}{12}$ 9. $3\frac{7}{15}$

Practice Set IV – 9

1. $\frac{11}{15}$ 3. $1\frac{1}{2}$ 5. $1\frac{21}{22}$ 7. $7\frac{1}{5}$ 9. $\frac{13}{20}$

Practice Set IV – 10

1. $\frac{1}{9}$ 3. $\frac{1}{20}$ 5. $\frac{49}{18} = 2\frac{13}{18}$

Practice Set IV – Chapter Review

1. $\frac{15}{17}$ 3. $1\frac{11}{16}$ 5. $\frac{3}{20}$ 7. $12\frac{43}{60}$ 9. $1\frac{71}{72}$ 11. 1
13. $7\frac{31}{60}$ 15. $\frac{23}{24}$ 17. $1\frac{1}{6}$ 19. $3\frac{11}{14}$ 21. $19\frac{11}{12}$ 23. 0

Chapter 5
Practice Set V – 1

1. 0.9 3. 0.25 5. 0.012 7. 0.5

Practice Set V – 2

1. 0.171875 3. 0.625 5. 0.25 7. 0.078125 9. 1.375
11. 0.75 13. 2.625 15. 1.140625

Practice Set V – 3

1. $\frac{3}{50}$ 3. $\frac{99}{200}$ 5. $\frac{63}{100}$ 7. $\frac{3}{10}$ 9. $1\frac{47}{250}$

Practice Set V – 4

1. 0.873	**3.** 0.778	**5.** 0.621	**7.** 0.65	**9.** 0.37	**11.** 0.43
13. 590	**15.** 1760	**17.** 1600	**19.** 1910	**21.** 1070	**23.** 50
25. 1430	**27.** 876900				

Practice Set V – 4

1. 25.108 **3.** 11.2615 **5.** 3.605 **7.** 22.506 **9.** 0.0883
11. 17.73 **13.** 2.8

Practice Set V – 5

1. 91.75 **3.** 10998.92 **5.** 9.2869 **7.** 0.0242

Chapter 6
Practice Set VI – 1

1. 1.40 **3.** 0.1414 **5.** 0.049764

Practice Set VI – 2

1. 105 **3.** 0.3216 **5.** 2388.33 **7.** 0.0066091 **9.** 800.46873
11. $148.48 **13.** $576.24 **15.** $27.90

Practice Set VI – 3

1. 36 **3.** 47 **5.** 2450

Practice Set VI – 4

1. 30 **3.** 150 **5.** 80

Practice Set VI – 5

1. 0.26 **3.** 0.058 **5.** 0.22 **7.** 3.01 **9.** 2.05

Practice Set VI – 6

1. 10891 **3.** 32.4 **5.** 64 **7.** 383.4 **9.** 100100
11. 80 **13.** 67.6

Practice Set VI – 7

1. 0.343	**3.** 34.3	**5.** 343	**7.** 3430	**9.** 3.43
11. 0.0343	**13.** 34300	**15.** 3.43	**17.** 0.00343	

Practice Set VI – 8 Review

1. 0.9828	**3.** 23.814	**5.** 39.6381	**7.** 1.2288	**9.** 2.02608
11. 0.13792	**13.** 10.76154	**15.** 15.65541	**17.** 13.08335	**19.** 5.74875
21. 5.25	**23.** 18.48	**25.** 60.7087	**27.** 1078	**29.** 1.4887
31. 0.0171				

1. 900	**3.** 2	**5.** 2.920	**7.** 0.041	**9.** 100.5
11. 9	**13.** 5	**15.** 20.2	**17.** 0.426	**19.** 0.098
21. 835.9	**23.** 540			

Practice Set VI – 9

1. 31420 **3.** 31.42 **5.** 0.3142 **7.** 0.03142 **9.** 0.003142

Practice Set VI – 10

1. 2310; 23.1 **3.** 48,236; 0.048236 **5.** 4691; 0.04691
7. 0.08569; 8,569,000 **9.** 187.54; 1.8754 **11.** 876,120; 0.87612
13. 0.0998; 9.98 **15.** 0.051; 510 **17.** 853,330; 0.0085333
19. 0.087632; 87632 **21.** 86432; 864.32 **23.** 0.087432; 87432

Practice Set VI – 11

1. 1×10^5 **3.** 1×10^6 **5.** 1×10^{-2} **7.** 1×10^{-10} **9.** 1×10^3
11. 1,000,000 **13.** 1000 **15.** 0.001
17. 0.01 **19.** 100

Practice Set VI – 12

1. 20,000 **3.** 0.0033 **5.** 0.0000000847 **7.** 8.39×10^{-4} **9.** 8,769,000,000
11. 0.0000006798 **13.** 3.57×10^{-3} **15.** 0.0000075 **17.** 40,000,000
19. 4.5789×10^4 **21.** 8.32467×10^3 **23.** 3.57×10^{-3} **25.** 1.0×10^{-5}

Fraction Review

1. $3\frac{25}{27}$ 3. $20\frac{1}{12}$ 5. $2\frac{21}{40}$ 7. $3\frac{1}{5}$ 9. $1\frac{1}{12}$
11. $9\frac{1}{3}$ 13. $4\frac{3}{4}$ 15. $3\frac{1}{2}$ 17. $6\frac{13}{32}$ 19. $\frac{7}{45}$
21. $\frac{66}{125}$ 23. $16\frac{4}{5}$ 25. $\frac{5}{18}$ 27. $\frac{3}{10}$ 29. $\frac{9}{10}$
31. $\frac{1}{2}$ 33. $812\frac{1}{2}$ 35. $3\frac{1}{5}$ 37. $\frac{3}{10}$ 39. $\frac{3}{10}$
41. $8\frac{1}{4}$ 43. $\frac{3}{4}$ 45. $\frac{4}{21}$ 47. $3\frac{9}{31}$ 49. $\frac{1}{2}$
51. $1\frac{13}{29}$

Chapter 7
Practice Set VII – 1

1. 0.15 3. 0.943 5. 0.09 7. 0.4 9. 0.05

Practice Set VII – 2

1. 10% 3. 90% 5. 76.2% 7. 12.5% 9. 8.5% 11. 225%

Practice Set VII – 3

1. $\frac{3}{5}$ 3. $\frac{11}{10} = 1\frac{1}{10}$ 5. $\frac{2}{25}$

Practice Set VII – 4

1. 25% 3. 83.3% 5. 18.8% 7. 70%

Practice Set VII – 5

1. 0.125 3. 0.5711 5. 0.095 7. 33% 9. 98.7% 11. 11%
13. 12.5% 15. 14.3% 17. 11.1% 19. 9.1% 21. $\frac{1}{50}$ 23. $\frac{1}{5}$
25. $\frac{8}{25}$ 27. $\frac{77}{200}$

	Fraction	Decimal	Percent
29.	$\frac{2}{25}$	0.08	8%
31.	$\frac{37}{40}$	0.925	92.5%
33.	$\frac{3}{7}$	0.429	42.9%
35.	650	650.00	65,000%
37.	$1\frac{1}{4}$	1.25	125%
39.	$\frac{333}{1000}$	0.333	33.3%
41.	$1\frac{5}{9}$	1.556	155.6%

Practice Set VII – 6

    1. 50   **3.** 500   **5.** 50   **7.** 75   **9.** 300   **11.** 30.006

Practice Set VII – 7

    1. $705   **3.** $465.80

Practice Set VII – 8

    1. 29.6%   **3.** 10%   **5.** 15.6%

Practice Set VII – 9

    1. $5.83   **3.** $5.28   **5.** $7.75

Practice Set VII – 10

    1. 4.48   **3.** 160   **5.** 112.7   **7.** 0.03   **9.** 307.5 sq ft; 1537.5 sq ft

Practice Set VII – 11

Item	Company A list price	Company A new price	Company B list price	Company B new price
general operating scissors	$6.10	**$4.76**	$4.45	**$4.78**
iris scissors	$7.05	**$5.50**	$5.00	**$5.38**
surgical cotton wadding	$4.20	**$3.28**	$3.85	**$4.14**
Needle holders	$4.25	**$3.32**	$3.00	**$3.23**
Endotracheal tubes	$2.38	**$1.86**	$1.93	**$2.07**

Practice Set VII – 12

1. 14 g% **3.** 0.9 g% **5.** 0.5 g% **7.** 1 g% **9.** 18 g/100 ml
11. 3.2 mg% **13.** 0.1 mg/100 ml

Practice Set VII – 13

1. 12 g% **3.** 8 g% **5.** 10 g% **7.** 0.9% **9.** 4.5% **11.** 2%
13. 70%

Chapter 8
Practice Set VIII – 1

1. 80:40 = 2:1 **3.** 12:5 **5.** 29:70

Practice Set VIII – 2

1. $\frac{1}{3} = 0.33$ **3.** $\frac{1}{3} = 0.33$ **5.** $\frac{1}{8} = 0.125$

Practice Set VIII – 3

1. $\frac{5\,g}{100\,ml} = \frac{1\,g}{20\,ml}$ **3.** $\frac{100\,mg}{1\,cc}$ **5.** $\frac{25\,mg}{1\,ml}$ **7.** $\frac{1\,cc}{5\,lbs}$

Practice Set VIII – 4

1. 20 **3.** 1.5 **5.** 40 **7.** 1000 **9.** 9 **11.** 0.4
13. 400 **15.** 0.01 or $\frac{1}{100}$ **17.** $171

Practice Set VIII – 5

1. 30 ml **3.** 0.4 cc

Chapter 8 Review

1. 1 **3.** 1 **5.** 1.125 **7.** 27 **9.** 1.5 **11.** 100
13. 10.769 **15.** 27 **17.** 15 **19.** 7 cc **21.** 13 cc **22.** 1.875 mg
23. 7 drops **25.** 5.5 ml **27.** 2.32 cc **29.** 9 g **31.** 17 mg **33.** 2.75 mg
35. 20 g **37.** 300 cc **39.** 4.8 drops **41.** 3.5 mg **43.** 32 mg **45.** 50 mg
47. 5 cc **49.** 0.52 ml **51.** 0.9 ml **53.** 0.36 cc **54.** 3.25 mg **55.** 4.2 cc
57. 0.4 ml

Chapter 9
Practice Set IX – 1

1. meniscus **3.** 1 g/cc **5.** 10.5

Practice Set IX – 2

1. hecto **3.** none **5.** milli **7.** centi

Practice Set IX – 3

1. dm; $1/10$ meters **3.** dkg; 10 grams **5.** dl; $1/10$ liters **7.** g; 1 gram
9. dg; $1/10$ g **11.** L; 1 liter **13.** hl; 100 L **15.** ml; $1/1000$ L

Practice Set IX – 4

1. 1200 **3.** 2100 **5.** 5510 **7.** 3000
9. 5,151,200 **11.** 0.112 **13.** 0.0123 **15.** 0.0235
17. 0.0034 **19.** 0.1511235

Practice Set IX – 5

1. 7   **3.** 12.7   **5.** 2.85   **7.** 1.59   **9.** 46.2   **11.** 908

Practice Set IX – 6

1. 104°F   **3.** 98.6°F   **5.** 0°C   **7.** 113°F   **9.** 37.8°C   **11.** –17.8°C
13. –40°F   **15.** –23.3°C   **17.** 77°F   **19.** –12.2°C

Practice Set IX – 7

1. 46.2   **3.** 2   **5.** 85.05   **7.** 1135   **9.** 592.5   **11.** 20
13. 3.55   **15.** 30.48   **17.** 1.59   **19.** 3.33   **21.** 45   **23.** 17
25. 3   **27.** 3.53   **29.** 200.2

Practice Set IX – 8

1. 2   **3.** 2   **5.** 40   **7.** 5   **9.** 6   **11.** 16.67
13. 1   **15.** 0.67   **17.** 1.06   **19.** 2.11   **21.** 12.68   **23.** 0.21
25. 3   **27.** 3.25   **29.** 2.4   **31.** 0.8   **33.** 1.59   **35.** 141.75
37. 60   **39.** 105

Practice Set IX – 9

1. 0.05   **3.** 1; 0.5; 474   **5.** 0.5   **7.** 250   **9.** 30   **11.** 15.4
13. 1   **15.** 180   **17.** 0.15   **19.** 4; 8; 16   **21.** 500   **23.** 0.25
25. 1500   **27.** 1   **29.** 30.8   **31.** 8

Practice Set IX – 10

1. pt   **3.** c   **5.** teaspoon   **7.** ounce   **9.** oz
11. gal   **13.** in   **15.** gr

Practice Set IX – 11

1. 10   **3.** 18   **5.** 10   **7.** 27   **9.** 108   **11.** 1312.5
13. 10560   **15.** 9

Selected Solutions 251

Practice Set IX – 12

    1. 1   **3.** 8; 4; 1   **5.** 1   **7.** 72   **9.** 0.58   **11.** 1.5
    13. 0.33   **15.** 60   **17.** 384

Chapter 10
Practice Set X – 1

    1. 5 cc   **3.** 160 mg   **5.** 6.25 cc

Practice Set X – 2

    1. 2.6 cc   **3.** 1.5 cc   **5.** 0.83 cc

Practice Set X – 3

    1. a. 3 cc   **b.** 13 cc   **3.a.** 0.6 cc   **b.** 2.6 cc   **5.** 1.4 ml   **7.a.** 187.5 mg
    b. 7.5 cc

Practice Set X – 4

    1. 1.4 cc   **3. a.** 2 cc   **b.** 3 cc   **c.** 24.3 cc   **d.** 11.7 cc   **e.** 6 cc
    5.a. 9 mg   **b.** 31.25 mg   **c.** 6.25 mg   **d.** 18.25 mg   **7.a.** 3.6 cc   **b.** 12.5 cc
    c. 2.5 cc   **d.** 7.3 cc

Practice Set X – 5

    1. a. 7 cc   **b.** 4.2 cc   **c.** 3.8 cc

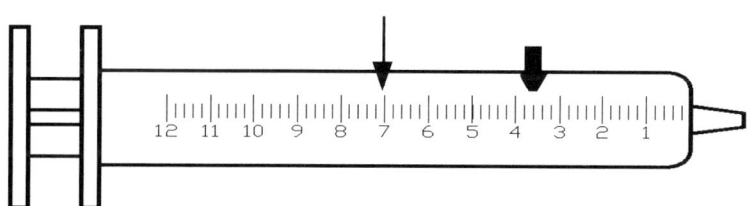

Practice Set X – 6

    1. 360 g   **3.** 25 g   **5.** 150 ml   **7.** 6 g Iodine; 12 g potassium iodine
    9. 2.25 g   **11.** 1 g

Selected Solutions

Practice Set X – 7

1. 22.5 g   3. 32.5 ml   5. 325 ml   7. 0.25 g   9. 20 g   11. 0.35 g or 350 mg   13. 0.9%   15. 5%   17. 3%

Practice Set X – 8

1. 3.8 cc   3. 0.45 cc   5. 1.2 ml   7. 1.5 cc   9. 2 cc   11. 18 g
13. 0.765 g or 765 mg   15. 0.95 g   17. 10.4 cc   19. 13.3 cc

Practice Set X – 9

1. 0.7 ml   3. 0.48 oz Electrosulf to make 1.5 gal medicated water
5. 11,000 ml = 11 L   7. 12 bolus/dose; 36 bolus for 6 days

Practice Set X – 10

1. a. 12.5 mg   b. 1.25 ml   3. a. 20 mg   b. 0.4 ml   c. 4 ml
5. a. 0.19 cc   b. 0.08 cc   7. a. 0.11 ml   b. 0.12 ml
9. a. i. 1.1 cc   ii. 1.54 cc   iii. 5.5 cc   b.i. 0.08 cc   ii. 0.06 cc   iii. 0.19 cc
c. i. 220 ml   ii. 154 ml   iii. 396 ml

Chapter 11
Practice Set XI – 1

1. 1.75 L + 0.75 L of diluent   3. 2.4 L formalin + 9.6 L H_2O
5. 2000 ml of 1% + 1980 ml H_2O 7. 2.1 L of 100% + 0.9 L diluent
9. 4200 ml of 5% + 3500 diluent   11. 4 L of 10% + 4 L of diluent

Practice Set XI – 2

1. a. 1.5 L 100% stock + 28.5 L diluent   b. 0.3 L of 100% stock + 29.7 L diluent
3. a. 5.7 L of stock + 0.3 L diluent   b. 6.6 L stock + 2.4 L diluent
5. 2.1 L of 100% stock solution + 0.9 L of diluent
7. 720 ml can be made by diluting what is on hand with 520 ml of H_2O.
9. a. 15 L of 10% + 15 L of H_2O b. 3 L of 10% + 27 L H_2O

Selected Solutions

Practice Set XI – 3

1. 700 ml of 100% needed
3. 3000 ml of 5% can be made
5. 2.5 L of 10% solution needed
7. 2500 ml of 2% sol can be made

Practice Set XI – 4

1. 1.4 gal of 100% stock sol needed
3. 1.5 L of 100% stock + 13.5 L H_2O
5. a. 1 L 100% stock + 19 L H_2O
5. b. 0.2 L 100% stock + 19.8 L H_2O
7. a. 4.7 L 95% stock + 0.3 L H_2O
7. b. 5.2 L of 95% stock + 1.8 L H_2O

Practice Set XI – 5

1. a. 1000 ml   b. 0.69 ml/min   c. 10.35 drips/min   d. 1.5 ml/min
3. a. 272.7 ml   b. 0.2 ml/min   c. 12 drips/min   d. 0.1 ml/min
5. a. 2090.9 ml b. 1.45 ml/min   c. 21.75 drips/min   d. 3.1 ml/min
7. a. 3818.2 ml b. 2.65 ml/min   c. 39.75 drips/min   d. 7 ml/min
9. a. 59090.9 ml b. 41 ml/min   c. 615 drips/min   d. 86.7 ml/min

Chapter 12
Practice Set XII – 1

1. A. 180   C. 170   E. 140
2. A. 2%   C. 6%
3. A. (1, 1)   C. (3.4, 0)   E. (4.6, –1.2)   G. (6.6, –3)   I. (8, 2.2)   J. (0.4, –0.6)

Chapter 13
Practice Set XIII – 1

1. 28   3. 190   5. 33.2   7. 630

Practice Set XIII – 2

1. True   3. True   5. c   7. b

Practice Set XIII – 3

3. $\bar{x} = 60.3\ kg$; $\tilde{x} = 61.5\ kg$; mode: 62 kg; range: 10 kg; $s^2 = 11.2222$; $s = 3.33$